With compliments

Knoll AG

experts in wound healing

knoll

W. Westerhof   W. Vanscheidt (Eds.)

Proteolytic Enzymes and Wound Healing

With Contributions by
M. Colonna, P. K. Das, L. Donati, H. P. Ehrlich, O. Estevez,
S. Garbin, J. Habraken, R. A. Hatz, E. Magliano,
J. R. Mekkes, T. J. Ryan, F. W. Schildberg, R. D. Sinclair,
W. Vanscheidt, M. W. F. van Leen, E. van Riet Paap,
N. C. S. von Jan, J. M. Weiss, W. Westerhof

With 35 Colored Figures

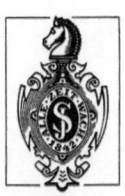

Springer-Verlag

Berlin Heidelberg New York
London Paris Tokyo
Hong Kong Barcelona
Budapest

Prof. Dr. W. Westerhof

Academic Medical Center
Department of Dermatology
University of Amsterdam
Meibergdreef 9

NL-1105 AZ Amsterdam

Priv.-Doz. Dr. W. Vanscheidt

Universitäts-Hautklinik
Hauptstr. 7

79104 Freiburg i. Br.

Springer-Verlag GmbH & Co. KG
Science Communication
Editing Dept. for Medicine
Dr. B. Fruhstorfer
U. Hilpert, S. Kempa, K. Kupfer, W. Rößling, Heidelberg

Cover: "Anatomy Lesson of Dr. Tulip" by Rembrandt,
© Stichting Vrienden van het Mauritshuis, The Hague

ISBN-13: 978-3-540-57816-1   e-ISBN-13: 978-3-642-78891-8
DOI: 10.1007/ 978-3-642-78891-8

Layout and Production Supervision: W. Bischoff, Heidelberg
Cover Design: W. Bischoff, Heidelberg
Typesetting: Schneider Druck GmbH, Rothenburg/T.
16 / 3130 – 5 4 3 2 1 0 – Printed on acid-free paper

This book is the fruit of lectures given during the symposium "Proteolytic Enzymes and Wound Healing" at the Joint Meeting of the Wound Healing Society and the European Tissue Repair Society held in Amsterdam, August 22–25, 1993. Looking back, we can conclude with satisfaction that the meeting was a great success, with regard to both the number of participants and the scientific level.

Enormous progress is being made in the field of wound healing and tissue repair. It was therefore of prime importance that one fundamental aspect in the healing of chronic wounds – the proteolytic débridement of tissue necrosis – be given thorough attention during the above-mentioned symposium. Renowned authors dealt with the various aspects of proteolytic enzymes and wound healing, so that a unique overview was given. The lectures were written up and arranged into the various chapters of this book, which should provide the reader with a practical guide in understanding and treating necrotic wounds.

Wiete Westerhof, M. D., Ph. D.

President of the Organizing Committee of the
Joint Meeting of the Wound Healing Society
and the European Tissue Repair Society

Contents

Pathobiology of Necrosis

P. K. Das[1,2], W. Westerhof[1]

Summary

Progression of wounds and their healing is very much dependent on the extent and types of necrosis, since the latter generally inhibits wound healing [1]. In this article we briefly outline the basic pathophysiology, classification, and immunology of the events which lead to necrosis. An understanding of the pathomechanism of necrosis is helpful in formulating the treatment modules in clinical management.

Pathomorphology and Definition

Sequential cellular death, usually recognized by light microscopy as eosinophilic deposition and bare matrix is often termed necrosis. In a pathology textbook, necrosis is defined as gradual morphological changes with the microscopic manifestation of cell death in a living tissue or organ, from progressive to degradative, due to enzymatic reactions on the lethally injured cells [2]. It should be noted that there is always a time lag between the identification of the events causing the lethal injury, the moment when cell death occurs, and the in vivo lytic activities. A brief description of the processes causing the changes of necrosis (from acute to chronic) is diagrammatically presented in Fig. 1. Generally speaking, two concurrent processes are principally responsible for necrosis: (a) enzymatic digestion of cells and (b) denaturation of protein. In the events leading to necrosis, particularly in skin, the stagnant blood lying in tortuous subepidermal capillaries is responsible for local anoxia and necrosis [3]. In this context, it should be mentioned that a somewhat distinct morphological pattern of cell death and subsequent elimination is termed "apoptosis" [4], further discussion of which is beyond the scope of this article.

Departments of [1]Dermatology and [2]Pathology (Experimental Dermatopathology Section), Academic Medical Center, University of Amsterdam, Meibergdreef 9, 1005 AZ Amsterdam

Fig. 1. Processes of necrosis.

Injury
↕
Manifestation of cell death

↓

| Autolysis | ↔ | action of enzymes: lysozomal and DNases of dead cells |
| Heterolysis | ↔ | action of secretory enzymes of recruited and inflammatory cells |

↓

Enzymatic digestion of cellular débris;
enzymatic digestion of surrounding matrix.
Denaturation of proteins/their deposition and digestion

↓ ↓

Table 1. Classification of necrosis.

Types of necrosis	Morphologic of appearance
Coagulation	Acidophilic opaque "tombstone"; loss of nucleus but with recognizable cellular outline and architecture often encountered during severe ischemia of heart and kidney. Such necrosis can also be seen in skin, as *black necrotic skin*.
Liquefaction	Focal appearance with lytic activity, and abcess formation, filled with white cells, commonly encountered in bacterial *infections* in brain and also in skin with yellow appearance.
Fatty	Chalky and opaque foci with shadowy outlines of necrotic fat cells surrounded by inflammatory cells, accompanied by the appearance in the tissue section of amorphous, granular, basophilis deposits; often encountered in acute pancreatitis. Such types of necrotic morphology can also be seen in skin with a yellow appearance.
Caseous	Appearance of soft friable and whitish-gray débris resembling clumped cheesy material with distinct granular débris and accompanying granulomatous inflammatory cells. This type is often seen in tissue infection, particularly lung with *Mycobacterium* and in skin with leprosy (erythema nodosum leprosum, skin tuberculosis).
Gangrenous	Histologic appearance shows combination of coagulative and liquefaction; often encountered in surgical clinical practice and most commonly seen in the lower leg, where blood supply is lost and bacterial infection with leukocytic infiltrates occurs.

Classification of Necrosis

Consequently, it is now well recognized that various pathways are involved in necrosis, depending on the homeostasis between proteolysis, coagulation/denaturation of protein, calcification, and the emergence of distinctive morphological types of necrosis. Histological recognition of the various types of necrosis, as listed in Table 1, is often helpful, first in recognizing the cause of tissue injury and second in designing the treatment modality [1].

Pathophysiological and Immunological Process

The immunopathological process of cell death is complicated and a detailed description of cell death leading to necrosis cannot be given here. Briefly, however, a continuum of progressive encroachment with feedback in normal cell functions is impaired as depicted in Fig. 2. In most instances of necrosis, normal tissue repair function is impaired either by internal en-

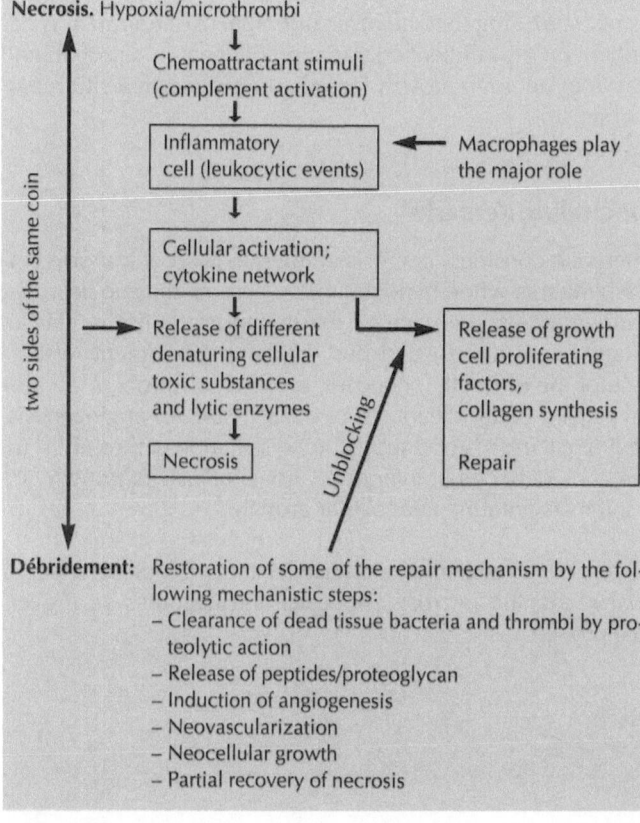

Fig. 2. Cyclic process of necrosis and débridement – two sides of the same coin.

Necrosis. Hypoxia/microthrombi
↓
Chemoattractant stimuli
(complement activation)
↓

| Inflammatory cell (leukocytic events) | ← Macrophages play the major role |

↓

| Cellular activation; cytokine network |

↓

Release of different denaturing cellular toxic substances and lytic enzymes → Release of growth cell proliferating factors, collagen synthesis
↓
| Necrosis | | Repair |

Unblocking

two sides of the same coin

Débridement: Restoration of some of the repair mechanism by the following mechanistic steps:
– Clearance of dead tissue bacteria and thrombi by proteolytic action
– Release of peptides/proteoglycan
– Induction of angiogenesis
– Neovascularization
– Neocellular growth
– Partial recovery of necrosis

3

dogenous causes or by exogenous stimuli such as infections. Adverse influences are hypoxia, trauma by physical and chemical agents, infectious agents, genetic derangements, nutritional imbalance, and, most importantly, immunological reactions. Microthrombus formation, hypoxia, and infections start the chain of events of "leucocytic infiltration", i.e., (a) margination, (b) adhesion, (c) emigration towards a chemoattractant stimulus such as complement activation, (d) frustrated phagocytic activity, (e) intracellular/extracellular degradation in the form of autolysis/heterolysis (see Fig. 1), via extracellular release of enzymatic products as well as cytokines from both dead and infiltrating cells.

In this context it must be emphasized that release of different lytic enzymes and denaturing cellular toxic substances lead to different types of necrosis, as depicted in Table 1. At this point macrophages play an important role, both as scavengers and in the débridment of necrotic tissues through the release of metaloproteinase; glycolytic/hydrolytic enzymes at the same time create an optimal environment for tissue repair. These cells also play a beneficial role by releasing various angiogenic and growth factors essential for healing of the necrotic sites. It is not surprising that the basic principal of débridment is dependent on the efficient degradation of denatured protein and release of de novo growth factors to restore the in situ repair mechanism.

Concluding Remarks

When one considers necrosis at the skin level, it is worth emphasizing that when hypoxia is the cause of chronic necrosis, as in leg ulcers, the necrotic tissue consists of fibrin, elastin, collagen, cell débris, and pus. Efficient débridment restores some of the normally occurring tissue-repair process via several steps, i.e., (a) clearance of dead tissue, (b) angiogenesis, providing a fresh blood supply, (c) dissolution of thrombus, (d) clearance of bacterial infection, and (e) release of growth factors, thus facilitating neocellular growth.

When such a restoration exercise (as the unblocking effect or repair) fails, the necrosis proceeds and becomes an irreversible process.

References

1. Westerhof W (1992) Pathophysiology of wound healing in venous leg ulcers. Phlebologie 21 : 77–82
2. Cotram RS, Kumar V, Robbins SL (1989) In: Robbins SL (ed) Pathologic
   basis of disease, 4th edn. WB Saunders, Philadelphia, pp 1–38
3. Wenner A et al (1980) Ultrastructural changes of capillaries in chronic
   venous insufficiency. Exp Cell Biol 48 : 1–14
4. Walker NI et al (1988) Patterns of cell death. In: Jasmin G (ed) Methods
   and achievements in experimental pathology. Karger, Basel, pp 18–44

Interview

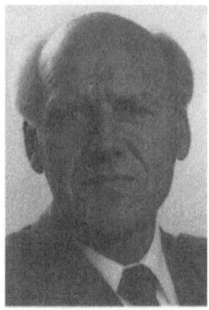

What do you consider is the most important aspect of necrosis?
Westerhof: It is often forgotten that there is always a time lag between the lethal injury, cell death and the in vivo lytic activities.

What is the most important pathway involved in necrosis?
Westerhof: There is never only one pathway involved. As a rule the type of necrosis is determined by a hitherto not fully understood homeostasis between proteolysis, coagulation, calcification and others.

Is there a common pathway by which the different adverse influences cause necrosis?
Westerhof: Very often we find microthrombi formation, hypoxia and secondary infections which accentuate the chain of leucocytic infiltration. Enzymatic products as well as cytokines are finally released from dead cells and infiltrating cells. Their extent modifies the morphological type of necrosis.

Types of Chronic Wounds: Indications for Enzymatic Débridement

R. D. Sinclair and T. J. Ryan

Summary

The role of proteolytic enzymes in wound healing can no longer be seen as mere wound débridement. Rather it should be considered as a single, but important player in the wound healing orchestra. Proteolytic enzymes are a family of proteins that serve to degrade necrotic débris derived from cell breakdown. They are produced endogenously often as precursor proteins whose activation is precisely regulated. These activated enzymes serve many functions in normal as well as pathological situations. In particular they are involved in the regulation of cell maturation and multiplication; collagen synthesis and turnover; cell deformation, migration and reepithelialisation; the development and removal of the perivascular fibrin cuffs found in venous insufficiency and leg ulceration, as well as the removal of dead tissues following inflammation. As a limited number of enzymes perform all these functions, it is difficult to predict the effects of applying synthetic proteolytic enzymes to a wound. Many such enzymes are currently commercially available and being promoted as alternatives to surgical wound débridement. It is important for their use to be considered in the context of their interaction with endogenous proteases, their physiological role in tissue, their ability to reach a desired target and the stage of wound healing at the time they are applied. Empirical observations and conventional wisdom however, support the view that sloughy wounds need to be débrided.

Introduction

Wound healing is often considered to consist of four stages that occur concurrently, namely: coagulation; inflammation,

Dr. R. D. Sinclair would like to acknowledge the support of Sandoz Australia, who have sponsored the Australasian College of Dermatologists Travelling Fellowship.
Department of Dermatology, The Churchill Hospital, Oxford, England.

clot digestion, fibroplasia and wound contraction; matrix formation and remodelling with angiogenesis and finally reepithelialisation (Table 1).

In using proteolytic enzymes to manage a wound, one must first understand the actions of endogenous enzymes and the mechanisms that activate and inhibit them, in order to comprehend the array of interactions exogenous substances may have. Many methods of enhancing proteolysis are now available to those involved in the care of wounds. Their main use at present is débridement of necrotic tissue from the wound bed and many find their effects variable and often disappointing. When an externally applied protease fails to achieve the anticipated effects, factors to be taken into account include failure to penetrate to the depths of the wound, inactivation or summation by bacteria, fibrin or fibrin degradation products or by other proteases. Chemical and physical factors, including fibre tension and temperature are also important.

Simply stated, proteolytic enzymes are proteins capable of hydrolysing peptide bonds. They can be classified as exopeptidases, which hydrolyse the amino or the carboxy terminal protein, or as endopeptidases, which degrade peptide bonds within the protein molecule (Table 2). Exopeptidases remove peptides individually or as pairs (dipeptidylpeptides), and endopeptidases can be broadly subclassified into three families according to the nature of the active site which may be a serine, histidine, aspartic and a fourth family if they contain a metallo molecule.

As our understanding of the functions of proteolytic enzymes has grown over the years, there has been an increased interest

Table 2. Proteolytic enzymes.

Proteins capable of hydrolysing peptide bonds.

Exopeptidases hydrolyse the amino or the carboxy terminal protein.
Endopeptidases degrade peptide bonds within the protein molecule.

Four families according to the nature of the active site:
serine, histidine, aspartic or a metallo molecule.

shown by wound healers in their other interactions in the wound healing process. These include the putative role of fibrin cuffs in the aetiology of leg ulcers as well as the role of the balance between collagenase and the naturally occurring inhibitors of collagenase such as the tissue inhibitor of metalloproteases (TIMP) in remodelling of collagen during wound repair.

Natural wound débridement in the initial phases of healing occurs through neutrophil derived elastase, collagenase, myeloperoxidase, acid hydrolase and intracellular and extracellular lysosyme. Bacteria also produce enzymes such as hyaluronidase that contribute to clot lysis and wound débridement. More recently, attention has focussed on another role of proteolytic enzymes, namely that of adhesion to factors such as fibronectin and the effect of lysis provoking agents such as plasminogen activator on epithelial cell migration, which is also a fundamental phenomenon in wound healing.

The interplay of all the above factors should be taken into account when judging the usefulness of a variety of proteolytic enzymes in removing slough and débriding wounds nonsurgically, such as have been used to remove eschars and to provide a suitable wound bed for skin grafting.

With the development of freely available proteolytic enzymes for wound dressings, interest is now being generated from clinicians as well as laboratory scientists who have made the empirical observations that these proteolytic enzymes are useful in making wounds heal faster.

It should be remembered that spread of enzymes in cellulitis and possibly also in wound healing can be through the lymphatic network. Entry into that network may be aided by guidance along dermal elastin fibres that are vulnerable to elastases. Exit from this network through desirable pathways also depends on the capacity of the lymphatics to respond to passive movement. This, too, depends on a functioning elastic network.

It is sometimes forgotten that the plentiful endogenous proteolytic enzymes, that so quickly decompose us after death, are the really important players in the wound healing orchestra, and that exogenous proteases used to augment the healing process interact at many different stages in the process. The way in which these exogenous agents influence the wound milieu will also be influenced by cell shape, intracellular protease inhibitors, and the by-products of wound breakdown. That healing is a dynamic process, and that the timing of these influences is equally as crucial as their mere presence, also needs to be considered.

Wound Débridement

The desire to remove slough from wounds and to débride them has moved in and out of fashion over the ages. Hippocrates advocated "scarification" of ulcers; however, with the late Middle Ages came the belief that laudable pus was a prerequisite for wound healing. Lister's influence led to a desire for antisepsis, and Gamgee introduced the absorbent and medicated surgical dressing to drain the "miasma" and to "-clean" the wound [1].

Exactly why débridement helps healing is more difficult to explain. One factor is that "Nature" abhors a space, and débris that occupies space prevents the apposition of healthy surfaces. It has been shown that devitalised tissue promotes bacterial growth. One suggestion was that in the presence of excessive bacterial proteolytic enzymes, fibrin is transformed into degradation products which are unable to support the migrating keratinocytes required for reepithelialisation [2]. Regardless of the mechanism, empirical observations and conventional wisdom support the view that there is a need to débride sloughy wounds.

Many agents are active in removing slough from wounds and have been used as an alternative to surgical débridement (Fig. 1). They have the advantage of being cheaper, simpler and more available than surgery, but until recently they did not rival the effectiveness of surgery.

The most ubiquitous non surgical débriders are the collagenases and proteases produced by colonizing bacteria [3] and the neutrophils recruited to combat them (Table 3). Recently the benefit of these organisms has been highlighted and it has

Fig. 1. Moderate fibrinolysis in the wound: a section of skin incubated on a film of fibrin showing lysis located over blood vessels.

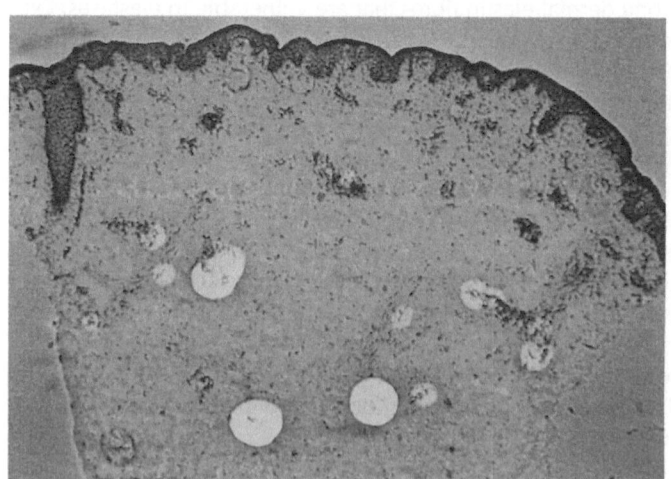

Table 3. Sources of proteolysis in wounds.

Neutrophils – elastase, collagenase, myeloperoxidase, acid hydrolase and lysosome.

Bacteria – many lytic enzymes including hyaluronidase.

Table 4. Therapeutic agents enhancing proteolysis.

Hydrocolloid dressings
Streptokinase with Streptodornase
Sutilains
Dextranomer
Stabilised crystalline trypsin
Plasmin and DNase
Bromelain (a proteinase from the stem of the pineapple plant)
Krill (a novel multi-enzyme preparation derived from Eupasia Superba)

been proposed that topical antimicrobials may delay separation of necrotic débris from the underlying wound and so delay healing. Other traditional methods include honey and sucrose, maggots, saline irrigation and wet to dry dressings changed frequently [4].

Agents specifically aimed at enhancing fibrinolysis (Table 4) include hydrocolloid dressings [5], aserbine, malatex, streptokinase with streptodornase [6], travase, debrisan, stabilised crystalline trypsin, plasmin and DNAase, bromelain [7] (a proteinase from the stem of the pineapple plant), and Krill [8], a novel multi-enzyme preparation derived from Euphasia superba, the antarctic krill. Some authors have even tried to augment their action with the carbon dioxide laser [9]. Perhaps the most widely used of these a commercial preparation obtained from the extracellular products of Streptococcus equsinulis that comes in a powder to be reconstituted with saline as a solution for use in dressings, or water and gels for direct application to wounds. It is a combination of two bioactive ingredients, streptokinase that complexes to plasminogen inducing a conformational change that exposes the active site and leads to activation of the patient's fibrinolytic system; and streptodornase that breaks down nucleoprotein emanating from dead cells [6].

Using bacterial by-products such as streptokinase/streptodornase begs the question of how bacteria in a wound influence healing. The mechanism of this interaction must depend on the mixes of bacteria and their products. So far these have not been subjected to study and consequently there are no reliable techniques to help us to assess their role in a particular ulcer. Another unexplored aspect of bacterial action is the host response. Intravenous injection of streptokinase for myo-cardial infarction induces deactivating antibodies but whether their presence in wounds induces a similar response and the effect of that response are not known.

While each approach and each enzyme has its supporters no single treatment stands ahead of the others in efficacy, except perhaps the hydrocolloid dressing that acts beneficially at so many different points in the wound-healing process that it may achieve near physiological proteolysis [5].

Computer Assisted Wound Evaluation

There has been a recent trend to use computer assisted analysis of wounds to determine their health. These computers describe wounds in terms of a colour code of black, yellow and red and use these colours to assess whether a particular wound is following the above programme or is in need of intervention to progress and heal. If the wound colour is assessed as black or yellow then surgical débridement and enzymatic reparations have been advocated, often without assessment of the state of health of the surrounding skin. In contrast, red is viewed as invariably good. This method is an oversimplification and it is important to consider the wound in a broader perspective before progressing to enzymatic débridement, which also interacts with the wound at many levels other than simply removing slough.

One can highlight the shortcomings of this method of wound assessment by considering the differential diagnosis of these colours. Deep red may be infected granulation tissue (Fig. 2). Yellow may be a thin fibrinous exudate, doing no harm whatsoever (unless incorrectly interpreted and acted upon).

Fig. 2. Sections from an experimental wound. Above: Thick eschar which impedes wound contraction and granulation tissue; below: thin eschar, the wound shows little contraction and adequate granulation tissue [5].

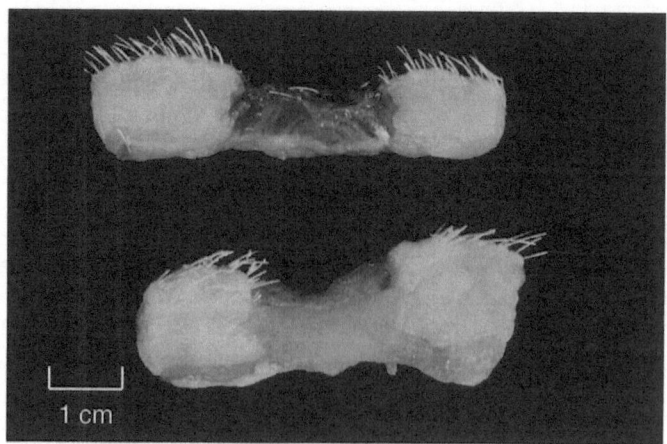

1 cm

The colour of the skin around the wound is perhaps as important as the colour within the wound. From it can be deduced the vascularity of the surrounding tissue, or the presence of pathology, such as contact dermatitis.

Accurate diagnosis of proteolytic bacteria such as Streptococcus or Mycobacterium ulcerans is important in the overall evaluation of an ulcer, however they are not necessarily associated with a detectable colour change. Odour is often a better guide. The use of a fluorescent light can be a useful aid. Anaerobic bacteria, such as Bacteroides melaninogenicus may produce a colour change visible with a Woods light but not to the naked or computerized eye.

While black eschars in the presence of adequate blood supply in the wound margins should be débrided, possibly surgically, this is visible to any observer. Red granulation tissue is itself an excellent débriding agent, but when it becomes infected, "proud" deep red or necrotic it is a barrier to healing and needs itself to be débrided. Yellow exudate is undesirable when thick, but the thin superficial fibrinous exudate can safely remain.

Fibrin Cuffs

Biopsies taken from the lower legs of patients with venous insufficiency appear to show increased numbers of capillaries. This apparent increase is due to elongation and increased tortuosity of the dermal capillary loops, rather than there being an actual increase in number [10], as is evidenced by the fall in capillary numbers seen on capillaroscopy of the dependent lower limb.

The alteration in the local capillary bed in response to calf pump failure is associated with increased capillary permeability, increased leakage of fibrinogen into the tissue and increased concentration of fibrinogen in the lymph. The pathogenesis of this fibrin leak has been postulated to be due to margination of white blood cells in slow flowing capillaries causing increased narrowing of the lumen and further slowing flow [12]. White cells so trapped in the capillaries degranulate and release proteolytic enzymes and superoxide radicals that damage endothelial cells [13]. Fibrinogen released into the tissues is converted into fibrin, which in the presence of inadequate tissue fibrinolysis [14], is deposited along with laminin, tenascin, fibronectin, collagen types I and III and various endothelial cell adhesion molecules [15] in a cuff around the outside of the vessel that can be seen on light microscopy.

These cuffs have also been shown to contain numerous growth factors, which may be sequestered by the fibrin present in the fibrin cuff [16].

In support of this theory that the pericapillary fibrin cuffs may trap growth factors and matrix materials which then become unavailable for tissue repair is the recent finding that despite the presence of these factors in tissue surrounding venous ulcers, venous ulcer wound fluid is unable to support in-vitro cell proliferation, whereas acute wound fluid is able to support proliferation due to growth factor activity [17].

This cuff was originally thought to act as a barrier to diffusion of oxygen and nutrition to the tissues that, in combination with the toxic products released by the marginated white blood cells leads to leg ulcers. However, it is more likely that the impaired oxygenation of the tissues occurs at a cellular level and is due to the increased diffusion distances that result from interstitial oedema, and that the effect of these cuffs is both to inhibit capillary sprouting and angiogenesis [15] and to interfere with the actions of growth factors. It also increases the stiffness of the vessel wall, preventing vasodilatation in response to the increased metabolic demands of wound healing.

Recent work taking sequential biopsies from the healing edge of ulcers [15] has shown that the disappearance of the fibrin cuff precedes the healing of the ulcer and can be hastened by the increase in fibrinolysis induced by compression bandaging [18], hydrocolloid dressings induced fibrinolysis [19], and fibrinolytic therapy with drugs such as the anabolic steroid stanozolol [20], phenformin and ethyloestenol (Fig. 3).

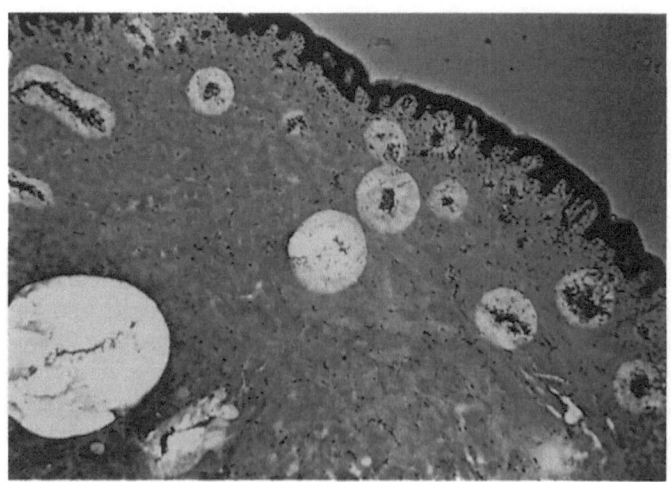

Fig. 3. Fibrinolysis occurring around each of the blood vessels in the upper dermis, shown by placing a frozen section on a film of fibrin.

Fibrin cuff lysis produced by these agents is not their sole mode of action in the promotion of wound healing and so it is difficult to quantify the importance of these fibrin cuffs in the aetiology of leg ulcers.

Elastase, Collagenase and TIMP

Collagenase is a metalloendoproteinase involved in the degradation of collagen in vivo. It exists in the skin in balance with a variety of natural inhibitors, the most important of which are called tissue inhibitors of metalloprotease (TIMPs). TIMP and collagenase are produced by normal keratinocytes as well as by dermal fibroblasts and can be demonstrated in cell culture from keratinocytes taken from the wound edge and from migrating keratinocytes [21].

As collagen synthesis is controlled at the level of transcription, further regulation outside the cell is controlled by the activation or increased production of collagenase [22], which normally exists in an inactivated state in the dermis in a 1:1 stoichiometric balance with TIMP.

Collagenase is involved in wound healing initially through clot débridement and in later stages through the remodelling of the collagen lattice into mature scar and finally in the termination of wound healing. During the stage of wound matrix formation and wound remodelling, collagenase, predominantly derived from macrophages and neutrophils removes old collagen to allow deposition of the new collagen. In excess this collagenase may disrupt the fibrin or fibronectin scaffold for epithelial migration and contribute to the failure of epithelialisation of some chronic wounds [3].

Elastic fibres in the skin generally persist for many years and turnover of elastin is slow [23]. However a portion of elastin is continually degraded and replaced, although less so with ageing. Elastases comprise a family of metalloproteases, the most powerful of which are derived from polymorphs.

Elastases effect wound development and healing in many ways. Firstly elastase induced disruption of vessel wall integrity plays a part in the development of varicose veins and venous hypertension [23]. Secondly, elastin in the dermis is intimately involved with the lymphatic network of the skin and disruption of the elastin by elastases disrupts the lymphatic system which is an important defence mechanism of the skin against the disruptive effects of proteolytic enzymes [24] (Fig. 4). Elastases are also involved in wound matrix formation in

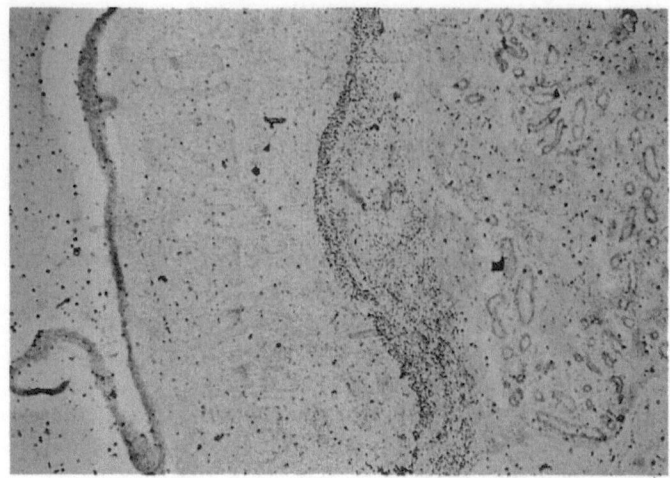

Fig. 4. Fibrinolysis only at the surface of the skin due to release of activators from epithelium.

disolving tissue elastin to make space for new collagen. Very little elastin is found in scar tissue and this is most likely a consequence of the abundant neutrophils found in the early stages of the healing wound.

Cell Shape and Proteolytic Enzymes

The interaction of mechanical stresses with the chemical environment in wounds is most easily demonstrated in the healing of bone or tendon injuries and in cosmonauts and paralysed people who develop osteoporosis after prolonged periods of weightlessness or immobility [25]. However skin has a similar constitution to bone and is also influenced by environmental factors [25]. External forces distort the cell cytoskeleton; these distortions influence the cell biochemistry and this mediates the cells response to its new environment [26].

The whole process also works in reverse so that biochemical signals can stimulate the cell to change shape, migrate, bind to another cell, prepare to undergo mitosis or to anchor to a basement membrane [25]. This is seen with the rounding of cells that occurs prior to mitosis [27, 28] and of endothelial cells in inflammatory states [29], and the changing shape of keratinocytes prior to migrating over the surface of an ulcer. Conversely fibroblasts elongate prior to initiating wound contraction [30].

The chemicals involved in mediating or responding to changes in cell shape include proteolytic enzymes and their inhibitors that antagonize cell adhesion and cytoskeletal resistance to deformity [28]. Proteases, if uninhibited, release the cytoskeleton from its attachment to the basement membrane or to solid elements within the extracellular matrix. Inhibitors of proteolytic enzymes act to reverse this [31].

Protein kinase C may act as a mechanoreceptor that when pushed or pulled phosphorolates vinculin [32] making it receptive to the attachment of the actin containing microfilament bundles of the cytoskeleton. Urokinase is an epidermal protease, which is co-localized with vinculin [33]. It can be visualised as clumps on the cell surface and it disrupts the attachment by vinculin and may act as a regulator of this system [25]. Protein kinase C is also the central regulator of a large number of intracellular chemical pathways, and so it is possible only to hypothesize about the net effect of mechanical distortion on cell behaviour, or the influence on or the regulation of this process by proteases.

Cell migration relies on separation of the cell from its anchors [25]. Collagenase, elastase and trypsin are capable of dissolving desmosomes and hemidesmosomes, which then enables the cells to migrate on a matrix of fibronectin [34]. Fibroblast and endothelial cell migration also require these proteases to enable them to move within the wound [25]. Termination of migration involves inhibition of these substances to allow readhesion of the cell to its new position in the wound.

It has been suggested that the migration of keratinocytes across the fibronectin matrix that occurs during reepithelialization may be influenced by the urokinase type of plasminogen activator (uPA) [35]. uPA has been found at the leading edge of migrating epithelial cells in culture and may act either to degrade cell débris into fragments that are chemotactic for keratinocytes [34] to clear débris from the path of the invading epithelial cells, or to direct the advancing edge of the cell.

Angiogenesis is the directional migration of new vessels into the wound and is a prerequisite for healing. Stimulation of angiogenesis is complex and involves the interaction of a number of growth factors [36], such as fibroblast growth factor (FGF), transforming growth factor (TGF) and epithelial growth factor, as well as a number of proteases such as plasmin and their interaction with inhibitors of proteolysis. Furthermore, the activity of certain growth factors is influenced by their interaction with molecules in the ground substance. An example of this is FGF, which is normally complexed with heparan sulfate in an inactive state and is released, and so activated by proteolytic enzymes. As previously stated, endothelial cells first migrate when released from their basement membrane under the influence of plasmin and subsequently anchor at the new site when the plasmin is countered by its inhibitor. As the tension in the fibre and the strength of its attachment determines its susceptibility to proteolysis, such proteolysis is likely to be maximally effective only when hydrostatic forces are dissipated or wound contraction is enfeebled.

Conclusion

Regardless of which product is used, there does seem to be a definite role for proteolytic enzymes in débridement of wounds to remove slough, decrease exudate and prepare the wound base for grafting. Correct timing of their use is essential, and, at present, clinical acumen is the better judge than computer colour analyses of when in the life of an ulcer to enhance débridement.

Most topical débriding agents do not penetrate to the depth of the wound, although hydrocolloid dressings can produce prolonged changes in the wound surface that indirectly cause deep as well as superficial proteolysis and débridement [12]. The overall role of applied proteases has to be considered in relation to the endogenous proteases present within the wound and the surrounding so-called normal tissues. Their impact on the wound healing process should be viewed in a perspective that incorporates the stage of healing of the wound and their ability to reach their target. These considerations rely more on clinical acumen and a large number of variable factors rather than merely on information about colour derived by sophisticated machines.

References

1. Elliot IMZ (1964) A short history of surgical dressings Pharmaceutical Press. London
2. Teh BT (1979) Why do Skin Grafts Fail? Plastic and Reconstructive Surg 63:323–332
3. Stone LL (1980) Bacterial débridement of the burn eschar: The in vivo activity of selected organisms. J Surg Res 29:83–92
4. Ryan TJ (1983) The management of leg ulcers. Oxford Medical Publishers. Oxford
5. Cherry GW, Cherry CA, Jones RL, et al (1988) Clinical experience with DuoDERM in venous ulcers and clot resolution in experimental full thickness wounds. In: Cederholm-Williams SA, Ryan TJ, Lydon MJ (eds) Fibrinolysis and angiogenesis in wound healing. Excerpta Medica, Princeton, pp 19–23
6. Carpenter BG, Hill SS (1993) Varidase (R) – the science behind the medicament. (Unpublished)
7. Ahle NW, Hamlet MP (1987) Enzymatic frostbite eschar débridement by bromelain. Ann Emerg Med 16:1063–1065

8. Westerhof W (1990) Prospective randomized study comparing the débriding effect of Krill enzymes and a non-enzymatic treatment in venous leg ulcers. Dermatologica 181 : 293–297

9. Tolstykh PI (1990) Characteristics of wound process after high energy laser débridement and enzyme treatment. Khirurgiia Mosk 6 : 12–16

10. Ryan TJ (1969) The epidermis and its blood supply in venous disorders of the legs. Trans St John's Hospital Dermatol Soc 59 : 51

11. Bollinger A, Speiser D, Haselbach P, Jager K (1988) Microangiopathy of mild and severe chronic venous incompetence studied by fluorescence videomicroscopy. Schweiz Med Wochensch

12. Thomas PRS, Nash GB, Dormandy JA (1988) White cell accumulation in dependant legs of patients with venous hypertension: a possible mechanism for trophic changes in the skin. Br Med J 296 : 1693–1695

13. Coleridge Smith, Thomas P, Scurr JH, Dormandy JA (1988) Causes of venous ulceration: a new hypothesis. Br Med J 296 : 1726–1727

14. Browse NL, Gray L, Jarrett PEM, et al (1977) Blood and vein wall fibrinolytic activity in health and vascular disease. Br Med J 274 : 478–481

15. Herrick SE, Sloan P, McGurk M, et al (1992) Sequential changes in histologic pattern and extracellular matrix deposition during the healing of chronic venous ulcers. Am J Path 141 : 1085–1095

16. Falanga V and Eaglestein WH (1993) The "trap" hypothesis of venous ulceration. Lancet 341 : 1006–1008

17. Salzman EW, McManama GP, Shapiro et al. (1987) Effect of optimization of haemodynamics on fibrinolytic activity and antithrombotic efficacy of external calf compression. Ann Surg 206 : 636–641

18. Mulder G, Jones R, Cederholm-Williams S, Cherry G, Ryan T (1992) Fibrin cuff lysis in chronic venous ulcers treated with a hydrocolloid dressing. International J Dermatol 32 : 1–8

19. Burnand KG, Clemenson G, Morland M, et al (1980) Venous lipodermatosclerosis: treatment by fibrinolytic enhancement and elastic stockings. Br Med J 1980 280 : 7–11

20. Petersen MJ, Woodley DT, Strickling GP, et al (1988) Constitutive production of procollagenase and tissue inhibitor of metalloprotienase by human keratinocytes in culture. J Invest Dermatol 92 : 156–159

21. Krane SM (1982) Collagenases and collagen degradation. J Invest Dermatol 79 : 83s–86s

22. Parish C (1986) Cutaneous elastin degradation in ageing and inflammation. Cosmetic Dermatology 1 : 97–112

23. Mortimer PS, Cherry GW, Jones RL, et al (1983) The importance of elastic fibres in skin lymphatics. Br J Dermatol 108 : 561–566

24. Ryan TJ (1989) Biochemical consequences of mechanical forces generated by distention and distortion. J Am Acad Dermatol 21 : 115–130

25. Ryan TJ (1985) The Dowling Oration: morphosis, occult forces and ectoplasm – the role of glues and proteolysis in skin disease. Clin Exp Dermatol 10 : 507–522

26. Curtis ASG, Seehar GM (1978) The control of cell division by tension or diffusion. Nature 274 : 52–53

27. Burger MM (1970) Proteolytic enzymes initiating cell division and escape from contact inhibition of growth. Nature 227 : 170–171

28. Nishioka K, Ryan TJ (1972) The influence of the epidermis and other tissues on blood vessel growth in the hamster cheek pouch. J Invest Dermatol 58 : 33–45

29. Gabbiani G, Hirshel BJ, Ryan GB, et al (1972) Granulation Tissue as a contractile organ. A study of structure and function. J Exp Med 135 : 719–734

30. Nishioka K, Ryan TJ (1971) Initiators and proactivators of fibrinolysis in human epidermis. Br J Dermatol 85:561–565
31. Singer II (1982) Association of fibronectin and vinculin with focal contacts and stress fibres in stationary hamster fibroblasts. J Cell Biol 92: 398–408
32. Hebert CA, Baker JB (1988) Linkage of Extracellular plasminogen activator to the fibroblast cytoskeleton colocalization of cell surface urokinase with vinculin. J Cell Biol 106:1241–1247
33. Morioka S, Lazarus GS, Jensen PJ (1987) Migrating keratinocytes express urokinase type plasminogen activator. J Invest Dermatol 88: 418–423
34. Lazarus GS, Schectler N, Jensen P, et al (1991) Proteinase metabolism in the human skin: The role of plasminogen activator and mast cell proteinases in cutaneous biology. In: Goldsmith LA. Physiology, Biochemistry, and Molecular Biology of the Skin. Second Edition. Oxford University Press, p 462–479
35. Arnold F and West D (1991) Angiogenesis in wound healing. Pharmacol Ther 52:407–422

Interview

What is your principal interest in wound healing at the present time?

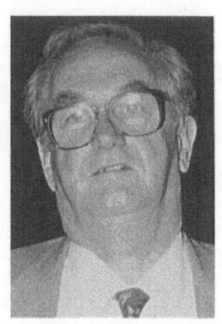

Ryan: The main problem is to get the available knowledge about wound treatment to general practitioners, nurses and the developing countries. Therefore, I have helped to set up regional training centres in Africa and Guatemala.

What is your point of view concerning treatment with proteolytic enzymes?

Ryan: When you try to use proteolytic enzymes on a wound you have to be aware of the role of proteolysis in general, which consists in remodelling of the tissue, cell movement, and all the functions of cell behaviour, including activation or inhibition of proteolysis. You have to bear in mind that the cells in the wound produce substances besides the enzymes you add.

What is the most interesting effect of proteolytic enzymes for you?

Ryan: Our whole skeleton depends on stable adhesions and on not being lysed. All balances between sticking and slipping are very important in the body. Proteases play a significant roll in that process. The cell that wants to stick has to prevent proteolysis by inhibitors.

Why Wounds Need to Be Débrided

H. P. Ehrlich

Summary

A number of factors are responsible for the great advances in burn care over the past 25 years. Aggressive fluid resuscitation followed by eschar excision and rapid wound closure are the clinical principles of modern burn care. The physiological state of burn patients improves rapidly after débridement and wound closure. Also, in the long run, the severity of scarring is reduced with early grafting. The disruption of the remodeling phase of wound repair seems to be related to the proliferative phase of repair and the cause for hypertrophic scarring. A therapy which optimizes the acute inflammatory response after burns promotes optimal wound closure and repair. The elimination of devitalized tissue in the wound bed creates an opportunity for the optimal inflammatory response to continue the promotion of the proliferative phase. Especially in patients with severe burn wounds, the removal of eschar by enzymatic débridement to promote rapid wound closure is cost-effective and reduces the added trauma of a surgical procedure and blood transfusions.

Introduction

The repair and restoration of damaged tissues is an essential biological process for the survival of the organism. The failure to adequately close a wound in some cases may jeopardize the well-being of the individual. The restoration of the skin barrier requires the regeneration of an intact epidermal surface and the deposition of a new subepidermal connective-tissue matrix. The type, degree, and severity of the trauma will dictate the magnitude of the repair process. The age, nutritional state, and overall health of the patient will influence the rate and quality of the repair. A young, healthy individual will sur-

Division of Pediatric Surgery, Pennsylvania State University Medical School, P.O.Box 850, Hershey, PA 17033

Fig. 1. Granulation tissue in a seven day polyvinyl alcohol storage subcutaneously implanted in a rat. The left side shows the proliferative phase of repair, the central area is the remodelling phase of repair and the right side is scar-like.

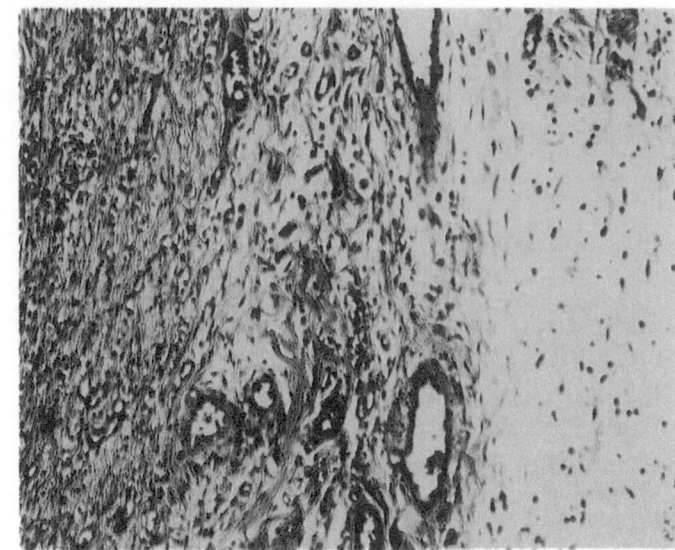

Fig. 2. Wound contraction in full excision wounds in a rabbit, over a 14-day period.

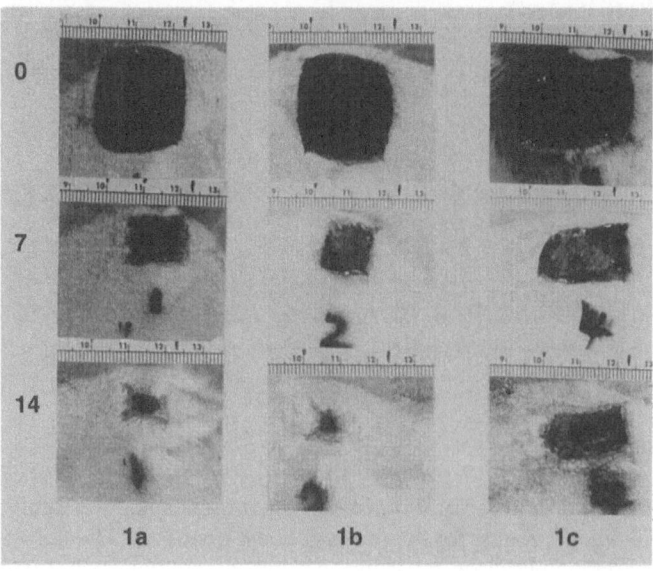

vive a severe burn injury, but often overheals and develops a hypertrophic scar. In contrast, an older individual or someone who is in poor health suffers a minor abrasion to the lower leg and may take many months to close that defect but shows minimal scarring.

Immediate closure of a skin defect by suturing or skin grafting will minimize the physiological strain on the patient. It appears that reducing the volume of the defect by incorporating viable tissue within it optimizes repair. In contrast, maintaining a volume of nonviable tissue within a defect retards repair and adds to the physiological stress on the patient. The complete removal of devitalized tissue maximizes the closure of sutured or skin-grafted skin defects. The presence of nonviable tissue in sutured or graft-closed wounds inhibits repair as well as promoting physiological stress.

With burns the importance of débridement is well illustrated. A number of factors are responsible for the great advances in burn care over the past 25 years. Severe burn trauma can cause death due to excessive fluid loss and rampant infection. Aggressive fluid resuscitation followed by eschar excision and rapid wound closure are the clinical principles of burn care today. The failure to achieve skin coverage by 3–7 days increases the risk of death [1]. There is an improvement in the overall physiological state of the burn patient shortly after eschar débridement and wound closure [2]. The clinical success of artificial skin grafting in burns is dependent upon the condition of the graft bed. Débridement of eschar as well as removal of newly deposited granulation tissue are required for the successful take of skin-substitute grafts [3]. The severity of scarring is reduced with early grafting. Scarring resulting from the healing of a burn wound depends upon how long the wound remains unclosed. In general, a delay of wound closure of more than 2 weeks will produce excessive scarring in a healthy individual [4].

The repair process is composed of a series of events which occur in sequence over a period of time. Initially, trauma produces an inflammatory response, which protects the host from micro-organism invasion. The early invading inflammatory cells such as neutrophils have a variety of ways to destroy such micro-organisms as bacteria. Inflammatory cells are important for the removal of devitalized tissue. Macrophage phagocytosis of necrotic cells and necrotic tissue is critical for débridement. A scab develops where nonviable tissue is separated from viable tissue. This separation of viable and nonviable tissues takes time and is dependent upon the acute inflammatory response. The success of the acute inflammatory response is related to the start of the proliferative phase of repair. Characteristic of this phase is the migration of other cells. The migration of epidermal cells over the surface of the defect is the process of epithelialization, which closes the defect. These cells migrate over a viable surface. The invasion of fibroblasts into the defect, accompanied by their increase in numbers by proliferation, populates the defect with cells which synthesize a new connective-tissue matrix. The nutrition of this new tissue is maintained by the process of angiogenesis, whereby new blood vessels and capillary beds grow into the newly de-

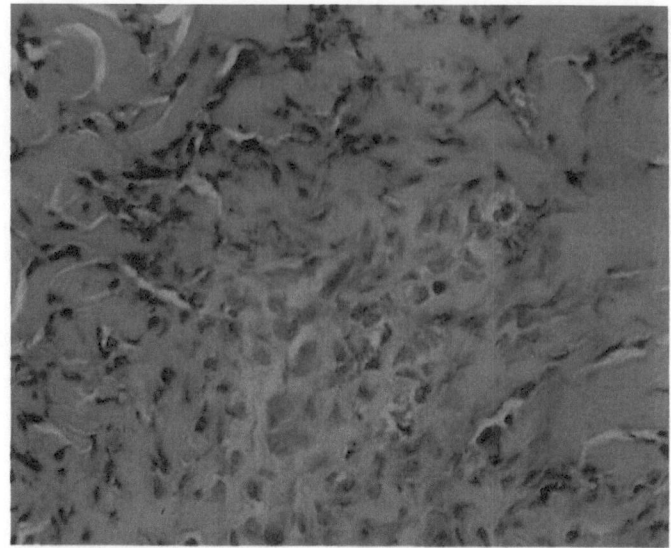

Fig. 3. Granulation tissue and surviving dermal fibers in a 10 day old liquid nitrogen freeze injury in a rat. This demonstrates that cell necrosis can occur in the absence of connective tissue destruction.

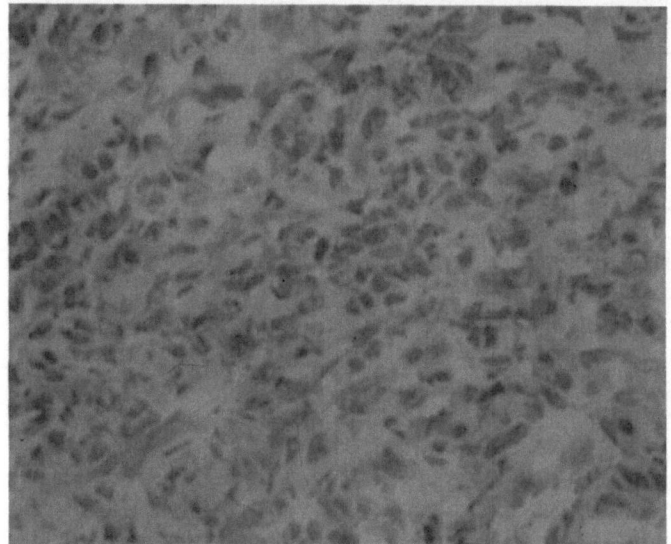

Fig. 4. Granulation tissue in a healing 10 day old burn wound in a rat. The burn defect losses both cell and connective tissue and a homogenous granulation tissue fills the wound.

posited connective-tissue matrix. The growth and integrity of this tissue increases as the new tissue matures. During the remodeling phase of repair a reduction in cell density and vascular perfusion occurs, but there is an increase in integrity of the connective tissue as the collagen fibers become thicker and more organized. The development of covalent cross-links within and between collagen fibrils adds to their insolubility and to the tensile strength of the newly deposited tissue.

Modifying the intensity or duration of the inflammatory response will affect the proliferative phase of repair, which in turn will alter the remodeling phase of repair. The disruption of the remodeling phase appears to be the cause of hypertrophic scarring [5]. The disruption of the remodeling phase of repair appears to be related to the proliferative phase, which can be related to the inflammatory response [4]. Prolonging or inhibiting the inflammatory response will lead to suboptimal repair. A chronic local wound infection will prolong the inflammatory response, which retards wound closure. Inhibiting inflammation with systemic glucocorticoids will inhibit healing [6]. There is an optimal inflammatory response for maximizing the quality of repair. A therapy or technique which optimizes the acute inflammatory response promotes wound closure and repair. Likewise, a condition or environment which impairs or prolongs the inflammatory response will reduce the quality of repair as well as increase the time necessary for wound closure.

The value and importance of débridement is related to optimizing the acute inflammatory response and the proliferative phase of repair. Open wounds can be a clinical problem, depending upon how they affect the well-being and physiological state of the patient. A chronic leg ulcer in an elderly patient or someone in poor nutritional health can take months to close and heal. Keeping such a wound from becoming infected and promoting its closure can be related to the presence or absence of devitalized tissue. A variety of dressings and techniques are employed to remove devitalized tissue. The continued appearance and accumulation of devitalized tissue within a chronic defect add to the delay in wound closure. Ongoing débriding therapy is needed to promote healing. A lapse in maintaining wound débridement in a chronic wound will retard progress in wound closure. In some cases acute débridement by surgical excision can jump-start the repair process. It may then be unnecessary to further débride such a surgically treated wound. The cost and resources needed for surgical débridement are high. Other techniques, such as special dressings, or additions, such as enzymes, may be more cost-effective, but are they as efficient as surgical excision? Chronic leg ulcers are rarely life threatening to the patient and skin grafting is not a common procedure for their closure.

Large burn injuries can be life threatening to the patient and aggressive procedures are needed for preparing a skin graft

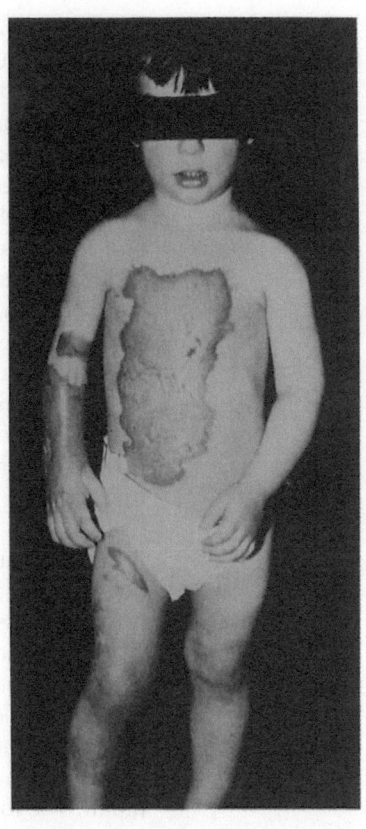

Fig. 5. Hypertrophic scars which developped in healed third degree burns in a young child.

bed. The débridement of the eschar from a deep burn is important. The use of topical antimicrobials will reduce the colonization of the devitalized burn eschar and allows time for autolytic separation of eschar and viable tissues to occur. This autolytic process is slow, variable in time for its completion and the patient is always at risk for infection and sepsis. The early removal of burn eschar, the site of bacterial colonization and wound infection, is important in severe burns. The complications of surgery and blood loss are acceptable in this clinical situation, because of the reduction in patient mortality with aggressive surgical excision. In patients with less severe burns the removal of eschar to promote rapid wound closure is still warranted. The possibility of using chemical or enzymatic débridement of burn eschar would be cost-effective and reduce the added trauma of a surgical procedure and blood transfusions.

Procedures and techniques that can rapidly and/or effectively remove devitalized tissue from an injury site can optimize the repair process. In slow-healing wounds the continued maintenance of a nonviable free wound bed is the desired state for closure of the defect. There are many variables which can alter repair. The elimination of devitalized tissue in the wound bed creates an environment in which an optimal inflammatory response can continue to promote the proliferative phase of repair. The local environment of a wound plays a critical role in its eventual closure and repair. Production of such an environment is the focus of this group of papers.

References

1. Shires GT, Black FA (1979) Consensus development conference: supportive therapy in burn care. J Trauma 19: 855–936
2. Echinard EC, Sajdel-Sulkowska E, Burke PA, Burke JF (1982) The beneficial effects of early excision on clinical response and thymic activity after burn injury. J Trauma 22:560–565
3. Jaksic T, Burke JF (1987) The use of artificial skin of burns. Ann Rev Med 38:107–117
4. Bauer BS, Parks DH, Larson DI (1977) The healing of burn wounds. Clin Plast Surg 4:389–403
5. Ehrlich HP, Kelley SF (1992) Hypertrophic scar: an interruption in the remodeling of repair. A laser Doppler blood-flow study. Plast Reconstr Surg 90:993–998
6. Sandberg N (1964) Time relationship between administration of cortisone and wound healing in rats. Acta Chir Scand 127:446–451

Interview

What are the main advantages of using enzymes to prepare a graft bed?

Ehrlich: The idea of using enzymes-like collagenases – is that they offer the opportunity of discriminating between viable tissue and dead tissue. This way you can preserve more viable tissue and have a better cosmetic effect. The idea of the future is to use an enzyme agent once and only once, and then to seal the wound with a graft. There is some preliminary evidence gained from animal experiments that collagenases will be able to do this.

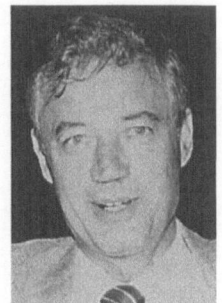

Why is it recommended that the eschar in a burn wound be removed as soon as possible?

Ehrlich: The necrotic tissue of the eschar does two things. It occupies space and it is a site of bacteria colonization. A graft bed that is infected with more than 100000 bacteria per gram of tissue will give a survival rate of only about 20% for the graft. If you have less infection, your survival rate increases to 80 or 90%.

What is your dream of future wound-healing facilities?

Ehrlich: The best-healing wounds are found in fetuses, and a fetus forms no granulation tissue, so the dream would be to heal a wound without granulation tissue, without the recruitment of too many inflammatory cells, thus reducing the amount of connective tissue produced and increasing the rate cover of the epidermis.

Surgical Versus Enzymatic Débridement

L. Donati[1], E. Magliano[2], M. Colonna[1], and S. Garbin[1]

Summary

Early surgical escharectomy has proven advantages in the treatment of extensive burns. It is justified mainly for extensive burns. The main indication for treatment with proteolytic enzymes is small (< 5 cm) second-degree burn wounds. Treatment with proteolytic enzymes is an alternative to early escharectomy in special cases: limited burns on the flexor surfaces of joints, hands, groin, heel, dorsal surface of the forefoot, and subunits of the face. Enhancement of the inflammatory phase of wound healing by proteolytic enzymes seems to be possible only in very early phases of wound healing. Treatment in this period results in a more rapid cleansing of burn wounds. Clinical experience has proved that the treatment of recipient sites by proteolytic enzymes leads to satisfying results concerning graft acceptance and later scar control.

Introduction

"Every wound has its own story." G. Sanvenero Rosselli

Tissue repair is fundamental to guarantee the survival of living organisms. It is a complex process involving vascular responses, cellular and chemotactic activities, release of chemical mediators, and biochemical and immunomodulatory interactions. Wound treatment and healing is an ancient art. Evidence of traumas and related consequences has been found by archeologists. In wound healing, the use of plants, biological fluids such as urine and blood, and animal products such as honey (but also pieces of fresh meat), mixed with folklore and magic, was common among ancient peoples.

It is amazing and fascinating to see that most of these practices are still in use: the ancient cultures gave a "healing hand" to

Institute of Plastic Surgery, University of Milan[1], Department of Microbiology[2], Niguarda Ca' Granda Hospital, Piazza Ospedale Maggiore, 3–20162-Milan, Italy the modern world. This interesting combination of historical and advanced knowledge helps us to better understand wound healing mechanisms and patient care [21].

Basic Aspects in Wound Healing

The wound is normally closed in layers. Each layer of tissue is repaired separately, approximating the wound edges, to allow healing by first intention. A large wound cannot be closed in this way, however. It has to be cleaned to allow granulation (healing by second intention). The latter is slower and results in formation of a scar, like a skin graft, which may be used to fill in the space and convert the healing process to first-intention healing. A third way to close a wound, sometimes known as tertiary healing, is the so-called delayed primary healing. Wound repair (Fig. 1) can be divided into three overlapping phases: (a) hemostasis and inflammation, (b) granulation tissue formation and re-epithelialization, and (c) matrix formation and remodeling. Inflammation is a progressive, interrelated event that occurs in response to tissue injury due to traumas. Soft-tissue trauma causes a mechanical disruption of blood and lymphatic vessels and immediate hemorrhage, fluid loss, cell death, and accessibility of the exposed tissues to bacteria. At the injury site there is firstly an immediate vasoconstriction, mediated by norepinephrine and serotonin, to slow down blood loss in the affected area. Almost immediately after injury leukocytes begin to adhere to the sticky endothelium of venules and capillaries. Just after neutrophilic margination, histamine is released from mast cells and platelets into the area and causes a further vasodilatation (cytokines-prostaglandines). Hemostatic and blood-coagulation mechanisms are activated in order to stop the hemorrhage (platelet agglutination, their entrapment in fibrin net, and release of PDGF, which stimulates the inflammation process and mitosis) [18].

The inflammation process goes on, leading to altered vascular permeability, extravasation of plasma components (albumin, proteins), aggregation of platelets, and activation of the coagulation and fibrinolytic cascades (acute phase – 15 days). Then the peripheral blood leukocytes (neutrophils) migrate via the circulation to the lesion, as a response to a variety of chemotactic agents and to regulate healing. Continuous activation of mononuclear cells gives rise to a chronic secretion of inflammatory cytokines, which amplify and promote the inflammation response itself (chronic phase). Leukocytes also release inflammatory mediators, which are necessary for the infiltration of monocytes. Later in the inflammation phase, the number of neutrophils decreases, while macrophages predo-

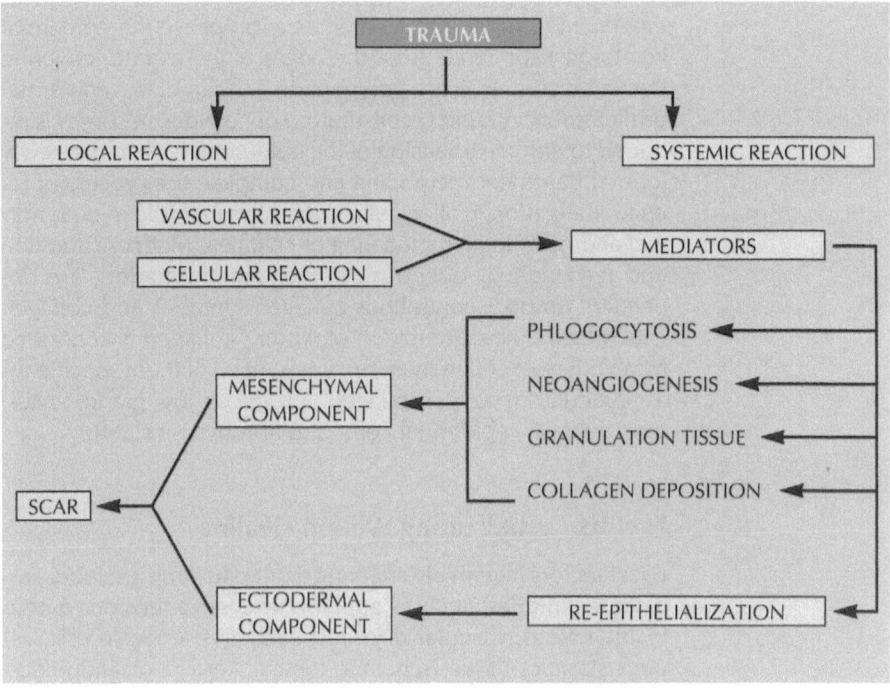

Fig. 1. Phases of wound repair.

minate. By means of chemotaxis, macrophages attract fibro-blasts, which in turn produce increasing amounts of collagen. A gel consisting of a matrix of collagen, hyaluronic acid, and fibronectin contains and modulates a newly formed vascular network (neoangiogenesis), to nourish the macrophages and fibroblasts that have migrated to the tissue gap. A consecutive increase of mitosis and cell replication occurs (mitotic phase). All the following elements take part in the granulation tissue phase: wound – matrix components – collagenases, glycosa-minoglycans, elastin, proteoglycans, type-III/I collagen, fibrin, fibronectin, hyaluronic acid; cellular components – endothe-lial cells, macrophages, fibroblasts, lymphocytes, platelets, epidermal cells [8].

The contraction phase is a muscle-like contraction of myofi-broblasts, a process that leads to wound healing after loss of tissue. The wound area closes up during contraction. This der-mal process can produce wound closure, with or without prior epithelialization. The myofibroblast is the most important mediator of this contractile process because of its ability to ex-tend and retract. Myofibroblasts contain one of the highest concentrations of microfilaments and actinomyosin [16].

The final result of contraction is a stable scar with a constant turnover of collagen and remodeling of the matrix (6–12 months). During the re-epithelialization phase the epidermal keratinocytes migrate from the edges of the wound, covering the entire area. EGF is a polypeptide that stimulates epidermal proliferation. A rapid reconstitution of hemidesmosomes is required to enforce adhesion of the epidermal cells to the newly formed basement membrane and complete the process of re-epithelialization. Collagenases play a crucial role in both normal and pathologic remodeling of collagen. Matrix maturation and remodeling, occurring during scar formation, are dependent on both continuous collagen synthesis and collagen catabolism. The degradation of wound collagen is controlled by a variety of collagenase enzymes, each of them specific for a particular type of collagen, produced by granulocytes, macrophages, epidermal cells, and fibroblasts [3, 24].

Factors Complicating Wound Healing

Local factors negatively affecting wound healing are: poor surgical techniques, such as applying excessive tension to nonviable tissues; vascular disorders such as arteriosclerosis, venous stasis or tissue ischemia; topical steroids or antibiotics; extravasation of antineoplastic drugs; hemostatic agents such as aluminum chloride or ferric sulfate, or alteration of the coagulation mechanisms with subsequent hematomas; venous sources of chronic traumas or foreign-body reactions; chronic radiation injury; neuropathic ulcers, decubitus ulcers, tumors (Marjolin's ulcer); adverse wound microenvironment (dry versus semiocclusive or photo-aged skin); and some topical antiseptics, which at high concentration are cytotoxic and inhibit tissue repair [2].

Systemic factors which may be bad for wound healing are: malnutrition, protein deprivation, deficiency of vitamins A, E, C, zinc, and copper; drugs like nonsteroideal anti-inflammatory antineoplastic agents, corticosteroids, anticoagulants, aspirin, heparin, nicotine; chronic debilitating illness (hepatic, cardiovascular, autoimmune, carcinomas, renal, hematopoietic); endocrine diseases (i.e., diabetes mellitus, Cushing's syndrome); connective tissue diseases; and old age (poor wound healing due to unknown reason) [22].

Wound Infection

As stated above many factors can affect wound healing, but bacterial infection is the most common and serious complication, particularly in burns (Table 1). Generally speaking, infection hinders wound healing by damaging tissue and promot-

Table 1. Definitions [4].

Infection: Microbial phenomenon, characterized by an inflammatory response to the presence of micro-organisms or the invasion of normally sterile host tissue by such organisms.

Bacteremia: The presence of viable bacteria in the blood.

Systemic inflammatory response syndrome: The systemic inflammatory response to a variety of severe clinical insults. The response is manifested by two or more of the following conditions:
Temperature >38°C or <36°C
Heart rate >90 beats/min
Respiratory rate >20 breaths/min or Pa CO <32 Torr (<4.3 kPA)
WBC >12000 cells/mm³, <4000 cells/mm³,
or >10% immature (band) forms.

Severe sepsis: Sepsis associated with organ dysfunction, hypoperfusion, or hypotension. Hypoperfusion and perfusion abnormalities may include, but are not limited to, lactic acidosis, oliguria, or an acute alteration in mental status.

Septic shock: Sepsis with hypotension, despite adequate fluid replacement, along with the presence of perfusion abnormalities that may include, but are not limited to, lactic acidosis, oliguria, or an acute alteration in mental status.
Patients who are receiving inotropic or vasopressor agents may not be hypotensive at the time that perfusion abnormalities are measued.

Hypotension: A systolic BP of >90 mmHg or a reduction of >40 mmHg from baseline in the absence of other causes for hypotension.

Multiple organ dysfunction syndrome: Presence of altered organ function in an acutely ill patient, such that homeostasis cannot be maintained without intervention.

ing excessive inflammation. Therefore, wound repair is delayed, leading to prolonged hospitalization and discomfort for the patient.

The mechanism used by micro-organisms to interfere with wound healing is correlated to collagen metabolism. Bacteria have been shown to decrease the synthesis of collagen and to increase its lysis, therefore reducing the collagen content of the wound. Moreover, bacteria lower the amount of oxygen available for the cells involved in the repair process, causing a delayed growth and migration of epithelial cells into the wound area, cellular necrosis, and microvascular thrombosis. These effects are due to toxins, enzymes, and waste excreted by bacteria into the wound environment, which destroy tissue and compromise the local and systemic ability to resist infection (Fig. 2) [11].

The term "micro-organism" includes viruses, chlamydia, rickettsia, mycoplasmata, fungi, and protozoa, as well as other

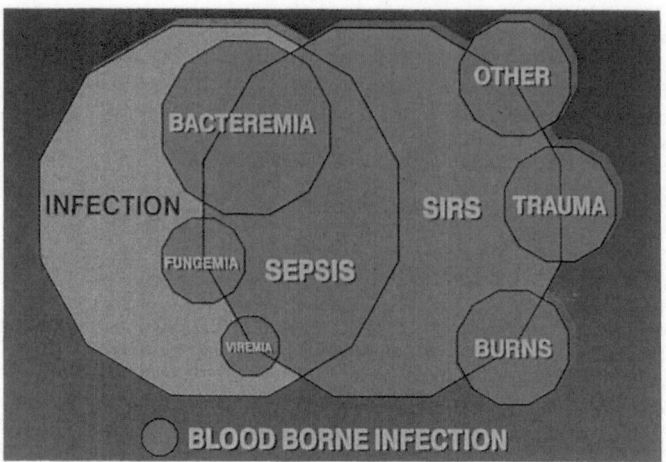

Fig. 2. The interrelationship between systemic inflammatory response syndrome (SIRS), sepsis and infection.

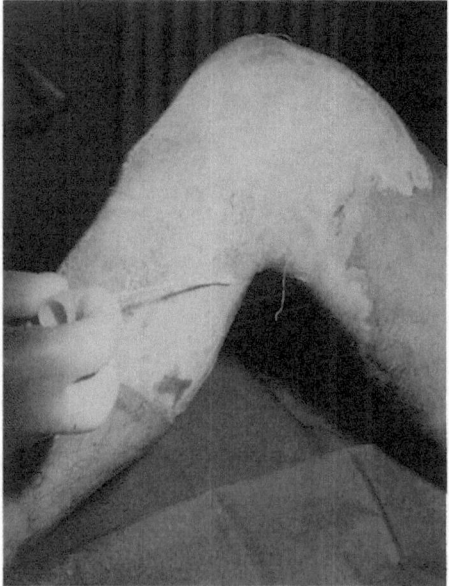

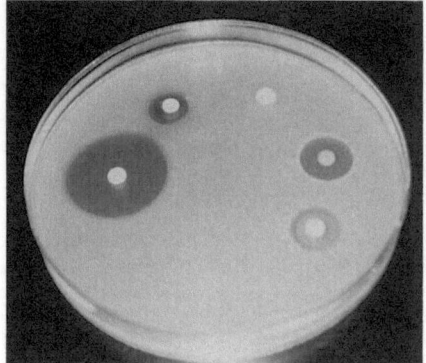

Fig. 4. Disk-diffusion antiseptic susceptibility (topogram) test on Staphylococcus Aureus; the zone around each filter-paper disk demonstrates inhibiton of the micro-organism by the antibiotic/antiseptic as it diffuses from the disk.

Fig. 3. Taking a swab from a deep burn of the right leg.

bacteria. Most of the wound infections are caused by endogenous organisms, particularly *Staphylococcus aureus* and *Pseudomonas aeruginosa* (also *Escherichia coli, Proteus, Enterobacter,* and *Klebsiella*) [7–11]. As soon as an infection is recognized, isolation of the infecting micro-organism must be performed in the microbiology laboratory. Moreover, the isolated bacteria undergo further evaluation for their susceptibility to antimicrobial agents in order to select an appropriate therapeutic agent. This must be done both for antibiotics (antibiogram) and for antiseptics (topogram). The factors involved in selecting the appropriate antimicrobial agent are: (a) the pharmacological properties of the drug; (b) the site and the seriousness of the infection process; (c) the general status of the host, including the immune status, usually depressed in burn patients; (d) the susceptibility of the infecting organisms [30].

In addition, we have developed a standardized method for defining the antibacterial activity of antiseptics in vitro. This method is an agar-disk diffusion technique employing paper disks with known concentrations of compounds. The efficacy of antiseptics is evaluated, according to the dimension of the area around the disks, as sensitive (S), resistant (R), or intermediate (I). Therefore, the antimicrobial therapy is normally based on the results of laboratory testing, identifying the bacterium and its antibiotic (parenteral) and antiseptic (topic) susceptibility pattern (Figs. 3 and 4) [15].

Basic Aspects of Tissue Repair Treatment

The first step in examining any patient with an open wound is to gather a complete history and make an accurate assessment (objective observation, determining location, shape, size, depth, temperature, color, margins, instrumental examination, diagnosis, and correction of the factor impairing healing). Once these contributory factors have been identified, treatment can be instituted [13].

Wounds must be protected from further damage, infections must be controlled, and débris must be removed. An optimal wound environment must be created to allow for rapid repair and regeneration.

Adequate hemocoagulation should be done if necessary (compression, torsion, electrocoagulation, suture). Hemostasis limits blood loss and the dissemination of microbes and toxins and limits edema, reducing pain and improving gas and solute exchange between blood and tissue.

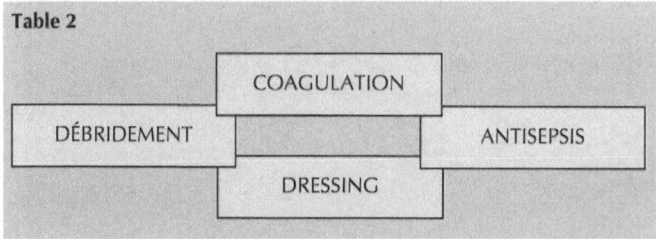

Table 2

COAGULATION

DÉBRIDEMENT   ANTISEPSIS

DRESSING

Blood and fluid drainage is also recommended. Optimal wound management depends on the nature of the wound. The purpose of dressing a wound is to accelerate (optimize) the epithelialization process. If left untreated, a scab will form, barring infection, and the wound will epithelialize under the scab. However, epithelialization does not occur as quickly under a scab as it does under a moist dressing. Both impregnated (antiseptic) and nonimpregnated gauze dressings are useful. An occlusive dressing also dries exudates. Covering a wound mimics the barrier function of the epithelium [10].

Antisepsis is necessary to decrease the bacterial count in wounds. Many active drugs can be utilized (Table 2). If a specific pathogenic bacterium is identified, the patient will be treated with the appropriate local antisepsis and systemic antibiosis. It is important to change the antimicrobial agents under the indication of repeated topograms and antibiograms, to avoid bacterial resistance and allergy phenomena [6].

The aim of the first antiseptic treatment is to remove débris. This can be executed by various methods:

1. Mechanical (sharp excision with scalpel, scissors, and forceps) (Fig. 3)
2. Physical (high-pressure irrigation, shower, water pick, tangential hydraulic forceps) (Fig. 5)
3. Chemical (with soaps, tensioactives, detergents)
4. Enzymatic (collagenases, proteases)
5. Surgical (knife, electric, or manual dermotome)

Débridement is the removal of necrotic and devitalized tissue from a wound. Five or six days after wounding, assuming a

Fig. 5. Tangential necrectomy.

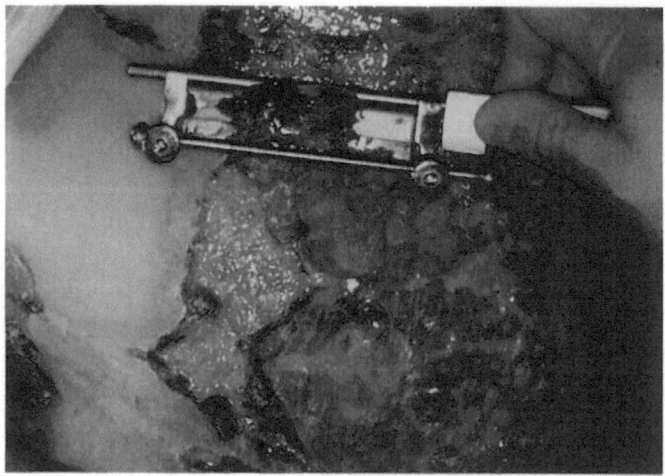

normal inflammatory response, macrophages derived from monocytes and phagocytic white blood cells (neutrophils) arrive at the wound site below the desiccated crust to complete the clean-up process. Macrophages that secrete proteolytic enzymes play a major role in phagocytic efficiency.

As macrophage débridement proceeds, these cells release chemotactic factors that attract more macrophages into the wound environment, along with stimulatory agents, which in turn increase fibroblastic proliferation and neoangiogenesis, leading to enhancement of the healing process.

In chronic wounds or in "complicated" wounds like burns, obstructive necrotic tissue (eschar) prevents the formation of granulation tissue and prevents epithelial cells from migrating across the wound. In wounds of this type, débridement removes not only dead tissue on which bacteria survive but also many of the micro-organisms that may be present. Bacteria and débris may be washed out by saline irrigation of the wound. When large amounts of necrotic tissue are present in a wound (as in third-degree burns), a combination of various methods may be used to speed up the débridement process and facilitate wound repair [27].

There are two main types of débridement: selective and nonselective. Selective débridement removes only necrotic tissue, whereas nonselective débridement indiscriminately removes both nonviable and viable tissue from the wound.

Mechanical débridement involves the use of scissors and forceps in an attempt to encourage eschar separation and removal of liquified eschar and exudate. It is often performed by experienced nurses and physical therapists under the supervision of the surgeon; it is usually done in conjunction with daily dressing changes and wound cleansing procedures. Extreme care must be taken to avoid removal of viable or newly formed tissue. Surgical débridement may be carried out down to the fascia or by tangential excision of a thin layer of the dermis down to freely bleeding viable tissue [3].

Common selective débridement may be performed in one of three ways: (a) with topical application of enzymes, (b) faciliating autolysis with synthetic dressing, or (c) by surgical excision.

Although selective débridement is the intent of the surgical approach, this method poses risks of sepsis and bleeding, owing of the trauma involving healthy tissues. Surgical débridement should be used with caution on patients affected by thrombocytopenia or coagulopathies or taking anticoagulant drugs. Its use is limited because of trauma, bleeding, or patient disappointment.

While this technique meets the principles of conversion of an open wound to a closed wound (grafting), it has been associated with extensive blood loss, limitating the amount of excision that can be carried out during a single procedure.

Débridement with topical enzymes is also selective, because enzymes digest only necrotic tissue (Table 3). When an excess quantity of wet eschar is present, proteolytic enzymes such as collagenases débride denatured proteins slowly but more efficiently in less than 15 days by attacking native collagen and peptides, as well as the fibrin dots and fibrinous exudates [9].

Moreover, in deep burns necrotic tissue may be anchored to the wound surface by chains of undenatured collagen. Collagenase can hydrolize undenatured collagen and facilitate débridement of necrotic collagen tissue [32].

Table 3. Fundamental collagenase properties for débridement.

- Selective site of action: not active on viable tissues
- Low antigenicity
- Capability to perform lysis of each type of eschar
- Capability through release of collagen catabolites to activate chemotaxis of marcorphages, lysomal autolysis, and cytokine release
- Capability to remove histones and to activate mitoses

In order to avoid denaturation and to maintain their activity, these substances must be mixed with water-soluble excipients, capable of transporting the enzyme close to its substrates.

Table 4. Advantages and disadvantages of the use of enzymes in débridement.

Advantages
- no need for surgical skill
- no bleeding
- rapid dissolution
- decreased hospitalization time
- ambulatory treatment is possible
- débridement is selective

Disadvantages
- cannot be applied on extensive lesions (more than 40% TBSA)
- possible interference and inactivation by common antiseptic drugs
- short acting

Most enzymatic ointments should be applied to the necrotic tissue every 3–5 h in very thin layers and then covered with saline-moistened gauze packing to absorb the liquified slough. When an excessive quantity of eschar is present the scab should be cross-hatched with a scalpel to allow the collagenolytic enzyme to permeate into it [25].

Autolytic débridement facilitated by occlusive dressing and in combination with surgical débridement relies upon normal phagocytic activity of white blood cells and is therefore the most selective form of débridement. Once débrided, a wound will normally undergo granulation contraction and epithelialization (Table 4) [3].

Factors Affecting Healing of a Burn Wound

The goal of burn wound care is to remove the eschar and to promote a rapid epithelialization of the partial-thickness injury or the development of adequate beds for skin grafting when full-thickness injury is present. Daily wound observation and care is mandatory [31].

Various approaches have been used to shorten the time of wound healing and to improve cosmetic and functional results. These techniques include combinations of topical drugs, débriding agents, use of biological dressings, and early excision of the eschar, followed by immediate autologous grafting if possible [14].

Burn wounds differ from other lesions in the following ways:

- They are rapidly colonized by potentially pathogenic bacteria (dead tissues are an excellent bacterial culture medium).
- They frequently contain large quantities of nonviable tissue, which remain in place usually for a prolonged period of time.
- They exude large quantities of water, serum, and blood.
- They remain open for extended periods of time.
- They frequently require tissue to be mobilized for their permanent healing [20].

Moreover, the avascular nature of the burn wound, secondary to thrombosis of vessels, limits the decreased endogenous immune response as well as the penetration of antibiotics administered parenterally. As granulation tissue develops and the eschar separates, exposed granulation tissue may be desiccated, resulting in secondary eschar formation. Bacterial invasion of otherwise healthy or partially injured tissue converts it to a full-thickness injury. Thus, the management of burn wounds is particularly complicated and requires all the resources of advanced wound care [26].

Clinical Applications

A clinical study has been performed in our department, using topical bacterial collagenase as a débriding and wound-healing agent for patients with burn wounds, diabetic and decubitus ulcers, and peripheral vascular diseases.

A combination of clostridiopeptidase A (60 U/100 g) and chloramphenicol 1% in ointment was used for enzymatic débridement.

From May 1992 to May 1993, a nonhomogeneous group of 120 patients was treated in our department. Among them, 90 presented with burns (TBSA 5%–30%); they were divided into three groups of 30 patients, treated with EEE (early enzymatic escharectomy), ESE (early surgical escharectomy) and ESE plus EEE, respectively. In the last case the collagenase ointment was used after surgery on the remnants of the necrotic tissue.

Thirty patients with ulcers (10 decubitus, 10 vascular, 10 diabetic) were treated with EEE. The patients were selected and divided into groups homogeneous for age, sex, and type of lesion (extension and deepness). Clinical paramenters evaluated included inflammation (clinical study: pain, erythema, swelling, warmth, functional impairment), healing times or times for grafts to take, and infection rate. Twenty-three patients with intermediate burns from the first two groups and six with chronic ulcers from the last group received keratinocyte allografts after the enzymatic débridement.

Results

Our results with clinical application of collagenase ointment have been very satisfying: significant acceleration of wound healing on the basis of enhanced granulation tissue formation and epithelialization were detected in each case.

Increased rates both healing and reduction of lesion size were detected in all the small burns and in all the vascular and decubitus ulcers.

In third-degree burns the graft-taking rate was higher (85%) with EEE treatment combined with ESE in comparison with EEE (< 65%) and ESE (> 80%) used separately (Fig. 6).

The infection rate was lowest with ESE (< 6%); this was followed by a good level of 10% with EEE plus ESE and finally < 15% for EEE (Fig. 7). Hypertrophic scarring and scar contrac-

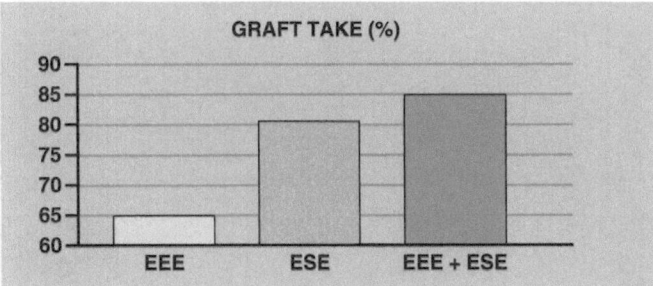

Fig. 6. Percentage of graft taking after EEE, ESE and EEE plus ESE.

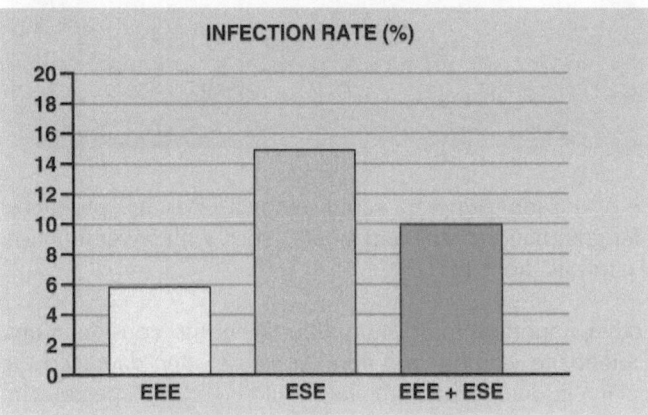

Fig. 7. Percentage of infection after EEE, ESE and EEE plus ESE.

tion were markedly reduced, especially in third-degree burns. Side effects, including local pain, scratching, burning, and erythema, were investigated: only a mild perilesional erythema was detected in three patients with vascular ulcers, but it disappeared within 48 h spontaneously [1].

On single aesthetic units and subunits of the face enzymes acted better than an early escharectomy or early dermabrasion, stimulating chemotaxis, phagocytosis, wound cleaning, and angiogenesis in blood-rich regions; in our experience, a limited and early débridement in these areas followed, if necessary and with specific indications, by elective surgical procedures, or vice-versa, and careful follow-up ensured formation of a normotrophic well-oriented granulation tissue and, secondarily, good-quality scar repair.

Moreover, we found that the effect of collagenase ointment on these specific sites was to enhance inflammation in the first moments of healing, resulting in a more rapid cleaning of the wound.

In critical areas rapid débridement is mandatory, i.e., of the flexor surfaces of joints, hand, groin, heel, and the dorsal sur-

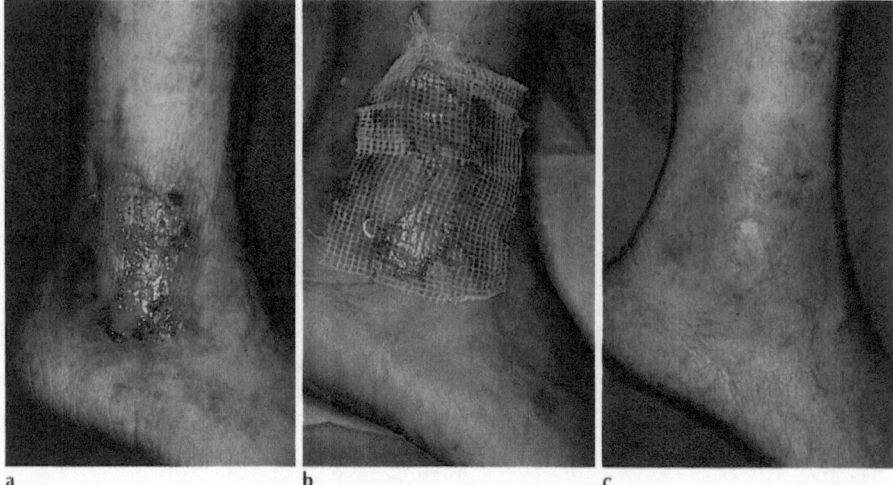

a   b   c

Fig. 8a–c. A Martorell ulcer of the lower third of the right lateral malleolus has been treated with enzymatic débridement and allogenic keratinocyte grafting with very good results in a short time (healing in 19 days).

face of the foot, where a rapid removal of eschar produces better granulation tissue and a better scar, with fewer functional complications [21].

Another important topic should be taken into consideration: recipient site viability and conditions are often damaged by local infections; eschar removal should be rapid, especially in case of signs of local infection. One should keep in mind that in these cases surgical necrectomy could induce both wound contamination and removal of viable tissues, inducing bad healing [31].

Thus, we can confirm that a combined treatment of the recipient site with enzymes can lead to satisfying results in cleaning, graft taking, and scar control, avoiding cytotoxicity, especially in burn wounds (Figs. 8a–c) [20].

Final Remarks

Since approximately 79% of the dry weight of both necrotic and living tissue consists of collagen, a débriding collagenolytic enzyme would seem to be an appropriate choice in wound débridement. Collagenolysis is well known to occur during normal wound healing, whereby a small amount of collagenase digests and remodels the destroyed collagen network.

Autolysis, on the other hand, is another well-known mechanism, mediated by lysosomal enzymes in the first steps of wound healing, beginning as a reactive process of self-débridement. This process can be enhanced – in order to obtain formation of granulation tissue and to accelerate healing time –

with repeated topical use of collagenases, exploiting the mechanisms of macrophage and fibroblast chemotaxis and activation by collagen-derived peptides, originated by bacterial collagenase within the wound.

Finally, collagenase ointment can be utilized as a valid, selective completion of different phases of wound treatment; we have performed and recommend the following protocol:

1. For all types of ulcers; débridement should be only enzymatic or a combination of enzymes before or after mechanical, physical, or moderately aggressive surgical necrectomy.

2. For third-degree burns, after the patient is admitted to a burn center, the following are necessary:
   – Complete escharectomy and skin autografting if possible;
   – Partial escharectomy and autografting, followed by collagenase treatment in case of critical graft taking;
   – Partial escharectomy and repeated treatments with collagenase, alternated with the use of temporarily artificial skin to prepare the recipient site;
   – Partial escharectomy and preparation of the recipient site with collagenases alternated with allogenic keratinocyte sheets.

3. For second-degree burns, during the time of eschar permanence, after admission to a burn center, dressing and antiseptic creams (silver sulfadiazine 1%) should be alternated with collagenase treatment for 1 week; subsequently, either débridement should be continued up to healing or surgery should be performed.

4. For superficial, second-degree burns, under ambulatory treatment, if the wound is not infected only application of collagenase ointment is necessary; if infected, 2 days with collagenases and 2 days with sulfadiazine.

Finally, we confirm that collagenase is an active agent for the removal of various types of eschar, including that formed in burns. It is most effective in promoting wound healing and tissue proliferation, and can thus be used to advantage in the treatment of various types of wounds. According to these data, we conclude that collagenases ought be added to the armamentarium of wound-healing treatment.

References

1. Abstracts of the 5th European Burn Association Congress, Brighton, September 20–23, 1993
2. Abstracts of the Joint Meeting of the Wound Healing Society and the European Tissue Repair Society, Amsterdam, August 22–25, 1993
3. Altemeier WA, Coith R, Cuthbertson W, Tytell A (1951) Enzymatic débridements of wounds. Ann Surg 134:581
4. American college of Chest Physicians/Society of critical Care Medicine Consensus Conference (1992) Definition for sepsis and organ failure and guidelines for the use of innovative therapies in sepsis. Crit Care Med 20
5. Barrett D, Klibanski A (1973) Collagenase débridement. Am J Nursing 73:849
6. Boyce ST, Holder IA (1993). Selection of topical antimicrobial agents for cultured skin for burns by combined assessment of cellular cytotoxicity and antimicrobial activity. Plast Reconstr Surg 92:493–500
7. Boyce ST, Greenhalgh DG, Housinger TA, et al (1993) Skin anatomy and antigen expression after burn wound closure with composite grafts of cultured skin cells and biopolymers. Plast Reconstr Surg 91:632
8. Cohen IK, Diegelmann RF, Lindblad WL (1992) Wound healing: biochemical and clinical aspects. W. B. Saunders, Philadelphia
9. Conell JF, Rousselott LM (1953) The use of proteolytic enzymes in the débridement of burn eschar. Surg Forum 4:422
10. Cooper ML, Boyce ST, Hansbrough JE (1990) Cytotoxicity to cultured human antimicrobial agents. J Surg Res 48:190
11. Damour O (1992) Cytotoxicity evaluation of antiseptics and antibiotics on cultured human fibroblasts and keratinocytes. Burns 18:479–485
12. Demling RH, Lalonde C (1989) Burn trauma. Thieme, New York
13. Donati L, Colonna M, Garbin S, Marazzi M (1993) Le Ferite e la Riparazione tessutale. Bi e Gi Editori, Verona
14. Donati L et al (1992) Clinical experience with keratinocyte grafts. Burns 18 [Suppl] 19
15. Donati L et al (1993) Infection and antibiotic therapy in 4000 burned patients treated in Milan, Italy, between 1976 and 1988. Burns 19:345–348
16. Gabbiani G et al (1972) Granulation tissue as a contractile organ. A study of structure and function. J Exp Med 135:719–734
17. Goldsmith LA (1991) Physiology, biochemistry and molecular biology of the skin, 2nd edn. Oxford University Press, Oxford
18. Hansbrough JF et al (1992) Clinical trials of a living dermal tissue replacement placed beneath meshed, split-thickness skin grafts on excised burn wounds. J Burn Care Rehabil 13:519–529
19. Howes EL (1972) Early investigation of the treatment of third-degree burns with collagenase. In: Mandl I (ed) Collagenase. Gordon and Breach, New York, pp 155–163
20. Kloth LC, Mc Cullock, Feedar JA (1990) Wound healing: alternatives in management. Davis, Philadelphia
21. Majno G (1975) The healing hand: man and wound in the ancient world. Harvard University Press, London
22. Mandl I (ed) (1972) Collagenase. Gordon and Breach, New York
23. Mandl I (1982) Bacterial collagenases and their clinical applications. Arzneimittelforschung Drug Res 32:1381
24. Moylan JA (1988) Trauma surgery. Lippincott, Philadelphia
25. Proceedings of the International Symposium on Wound Management, Helsingor, May 27–28, 1991

26. Proceedings of the 25th American Burn Association Congress, Cincinnati, March 24–27, 1993
27. Signorini M, Grappolini S, Magliano E, et al (1992) Updated evaluation of the activity of antibiotics in a burn center. Burns 18:500–503
28. Teepe RGC (1993) Cultured keratinocyte grafting: implications for wound healing. Elsevier, Amsterdam
29. Zimmermann WE (1972) The importance of collagenase for the local treatment of major burns. In: Mandl I (ed) Collagenase. Gordon and Breach, New York, pp 131–141

Interview

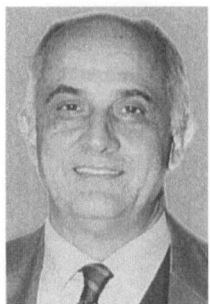

What is the main focus of your clinical work?

Donati: In our department we have a close cooperation between the surgeons and biologists. Cultivating keratinocytes on carriers to be used as artificial skin in patients with extensive burns has been among the main interests of our lab.

What should doctors know, who work with enzymes on wounds?

Donati: It is important that clinical doctors be aware of the fact that other preparations that are used in the treatment of burns can influence the activity of the enzymes. We found that the antiseptic silver-nitrate 5% inactivates collagenase. Other antiseptics, like mercurochrome, have a negative influence on cultured keratinocytes.

What is your treatment of choice for eschar in burn wounds?

Donati: In our department we have found it useful to combine a moderately aggressive surgical necrotomy with subsequent collagenase treatment.

Evaluation of Wound Débridement Using Computerized Image Analysis

J. R. Mekkes[1], W. Westerhof[1], E. van Riet Paap[2], J. Habraken[2], and O. Estevez[2]

Summary

A new digital image analysis (DIA) system was developed, which allows quantification of the débriding properties of wound-care products. The system consists of a videocamera with zoom lens, filters to eliminate reflections, an AT-386 computer, a frame grabber, two color monitors, and a digitizing tablet. Its main advantages are that the quality of the image can be checked immediately; bed-side measurements are possible. The measurements by DIA proved to be accurate and reproducible. Therefore, it can be used for observer-blind and double-blind clinical multicenter studies. In future studies, all wound-care products should be evaluated with an observer-blind, quantitative system like DIA.

Introduction

The process of wound healing is usually divided into four different phases: débridement, granulation tissue formation, epithelialization, and remodeling. Wound cleaning (débridement) is an essential first phase in wound healing [1]. Specialized phagocytic cells and even fibroblasts and keratinocytes digest the tissue components using natural proteolytic enzymes such as collagenase, thrombin, plasmin, chymotrypsin-like enzymes, and metalloproteinases [2–8]. Subsequently, the defective tissue is invaded and replaced by granulation tissue, and later covered by the epidermis. Finally, remodeling of the dermal tissues starts, which may lead to unwanted contraction and scar formation.

All phases, but especially the first three, can be accelerated or otherwise improved by local wound-care products or systemic drugs. The clinician can choose from an overwhelming range of wound-care products. Some of these products, like

Academisch Medisch Centrum, [1]Department of Dermatology, [2]Department of Medical Physics, Meibergdreef 9, 1105 AZ Amsterdam, The Netherlands saline-soaked gauzes, proteolytic enzymes, hydrocolloid dressings, dextranomers, or intracavity gels, are suitable for wound cleaning [2, 9]. One single product is not suitable for all phases of wound healing. For instance, it would be unwise and unethical to use proteolytic enzymes, designed for wound cleaning, in a clean, granulating wound in which epithelialization starts.

To perform clinical trials of wound-care products or treatment procedures, quantitative and objective methods for the evaluation of wound repair are essential. Different evaluation techniques may be required for different phases. Also the wound type and the kind of product to be evaluated determine which evaluation method is appropriate. In deep wounds like decubitus ulcers one may want to measure how fast the wound fills up with granulation tissue. In this case, volume is an important parameter. Stereophotogrammetry can be used [10], but it cannot be applied in wounds with undermined borders. Calculating the volume by casting, or filling it up with water, is an alternative [11–14]. These volumetric methods may be unreliable, as the volume of some wounds changes tremendously depending on the position of the patient. In addition, casting may be painful. Recently, some promising new noninvasive volumetric techniques using ultrasonic imaging, laser profilometry, or color-coded structured light have been described [15–17].

In superficial wounds like venous leg ulcers, volume is not an important parameter. In these wounds we are interested in the daily changes in wound size and in the color changes reflecting the shift from yellow necrotic tissue to healthy red granulation tissue during wound healing. The wound surface is easy to calculate from wound margin tracings on a transparent sheet; if necessary, a computer system can be used for calculations.

Wound contraction is not easy to quantify in a clinical situation. One needs orientation marks like moles to be able to measure the approximation of the wound edges. In animal studies tattoos can be used. Scar formation and fibrosis are difficult to quantify, apart from using invasive histological techniques.

Measuring Wound Débridement

To study the effect of wound-care products designed for débridement, the wound size or the time until wound closure should not be used as an end-point criterium, since they are influenced by a cascade of events taking place after the débridement phase. The débriding effect is usually quantified using the black-yellow-red system, in which black is black necrosis, yellow is yellow necrosis (slough), and red is granulation tissue [18]. This system has been generally accepted by clinicians as a tool to classify wounds on the basis of color. Some pharmaceutical companies have grouped their wound-care products according to the same classification model.

In clinical studies of débriding agents, until now only visual estimations of the area covered with necrosis or granulation tissue have been used. The red granulating wound area is clearly distinguishable by the human eye but, because of the complex two-dimensional structure, difficult to estimate.

Visual estimations of the amount of granulation tissue in a wound are usually unreliable, subjective, and not reproducible, although the experienced observer may estimate the surface quite accurately. We have developed a new digital image analysis (DIA) system which can measure the shift from black/yellow necrosis to red granulation tissue objectively.

Methods

A video image of an ulcer is obtained by positioning a video camera and a light source, both mounted with polaroid filters, in a standardized way to the wound. All variables such as height, distance, angle, light, diaphragm, etc. are recorded. The zoom lens adapts to any wound size. Ink marks are made on the adjacent skin to facilitate positioning. The distances between three of these marks are recorded for calibration purposes. The video image can be projected on the image stored the day before, to get exactly the same close-up. A color scale and a gray scale can be positioned near the wound for calibration purposes.

Hardware

The computer system consists of an IBM-compatible AT-386 personal computer, a frame grabber, a VGA monitor and an RGB monitor, and a digitizing tablet (Fig. 1). Since each stored image requires 500 kb, two large hard disks and a tape streamer are installed.

Software

The software was specially written by the department of Medical Physics of the Academisch Medisch Centrum and consists

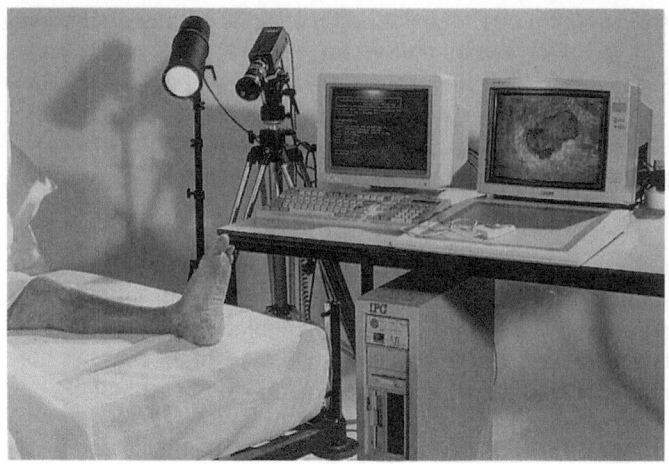

Fig.1. The DIA system consists of an AT-386 personal computer provided with a frame grabber, a VGA and an RGB monitor, a digitizing tablet, a video camera mounted with a zoom lens and polaroid filter, and a light source.

of a mixture of the original software provided with the frame grabber, programs written in the language C, and a menu structure composed of MS-DOS batchfiles.

Calibration Procedures

In the video system each color is composed of a certain amount (divided into 32 steps) of red, green, and blue light. In total, the computer system can recognize 32768 different colors. The computer has to be told which colors can be encountered in the granulating area or necrotic area of a leg ulcer. A labeling system classifying certain colors as débris or granulation tissue is generated semiautomatically by the computer, based on a large number of small representative wound areas selected from the computer screen by the clinician. The colors found in these spots are combined and stored in a color knowledge base. The system can measure and correct for color deviations and light conditions. Every part of the computer image can be enlarged if necessary for calibration purposes. The color of each individual pixel encountered in a certain area can be determined. Analyzed images and measurement results can be stored.

Measurement Procedures

After reloading of the stored image, the ulcer outline is traced on the screen using the digitizing tablet. After entering the horizontal and vertical distances between the ink marks into the computer, the red, yellow, black, and total wound areas are calculated, in pixels, percentages, and square millimeters. It takes about 2 min to fully measure one wound.

Results

Figure 2 (photographed directly from the computer monitor) shows a typical venous leg ulcer. The red granulating wound area is clearly distinguishable but, because of the complex two-dimensional structure, difficult to estimate. Figure 3 shows how the areas are recognized by the computer system. Depending on the quality of the image (reflections), and contaminations (textile fibers, zinc ointment, etc.) in the ulcer, a certain amount (0.01–5%) of the surface remains unclassified. The system has been used in clinical human trials and in animal studies (pig) [9]. In the animal study, the amount of unclassified wound area was between 0.01 and 0.3%. In this study, the amount of granulation tissue in the ulcers, estimated

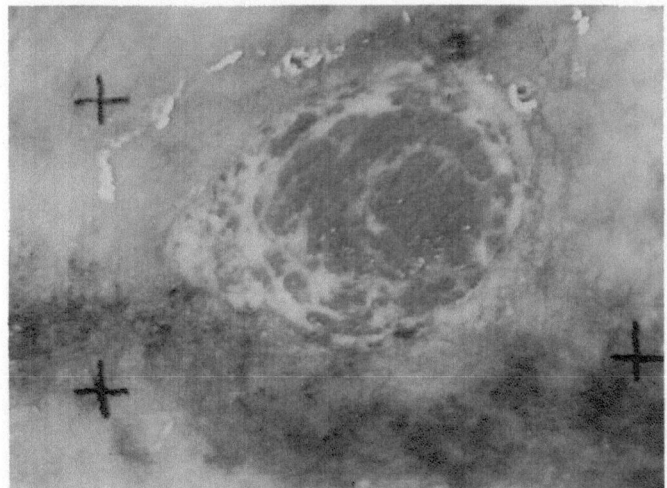

Fig. 2. Digitalized image of a venous leg ulcer (photographed from monitor).

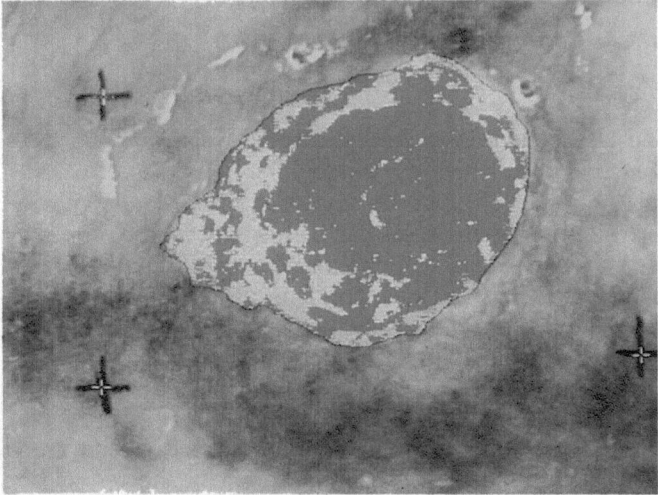

Fig. 3. The same ulcer as in Fig. 2, analyzed by the computer system. (*Red,* granulation tissue; *yellow,* yellow necrosis; *blue-black necrosis; white,* unclassified).

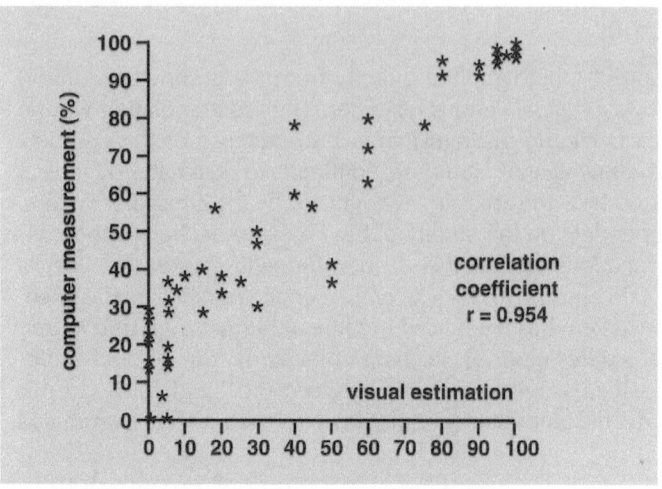

Fig. 4. The correlation between the amount of granulation tissue estimated visually and by computer image analysis in 64 experimental animal wounds.

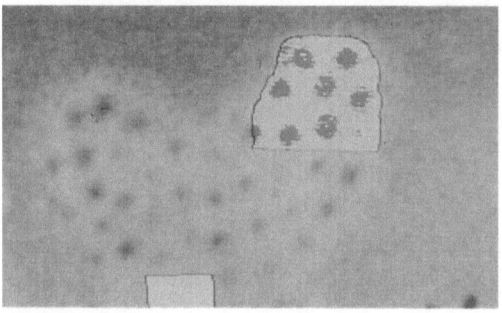

Fig. 5. A vitiligo lesion, under treatment with a skin-grafting method. The right part of the lesion has been analyzed with the DIA system to measure the repigmented area.

visually by an experienced observer, was compared with the computer measurements (Fig. 4). The correlation between the two methods was good ($r = 0.954$), but it appeared that small amounts of granulation tissue (below 20%) in an ulcer are underestimated by the human observer.

Discussion

The DIA system described above is a reliable and simple method for quantifying the débriding properties of wound-care products [19]. The advantages of this system compared with similar systems described before [20] are the possibility of checking the quality of the image immediately and of performing bed-side measurements if necessary, the absence of a photographic step, the possibility of obtaining exactly the same close-up, the flexibility regarding wound size, and the complete elimination of reflection by means of two polaroid filters.

The measurements made by the computer are accurate and reproducible. For a good interpretation of the results one

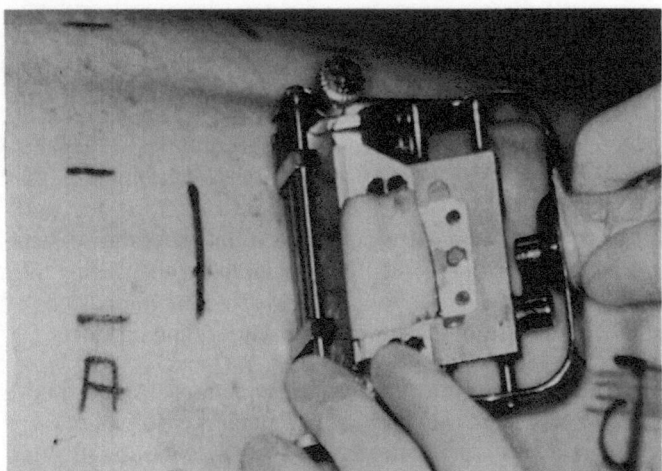

Fig. 6. An example of an animal study: 2.5 mm of skin is excised using a Brown electrical Dermatome.

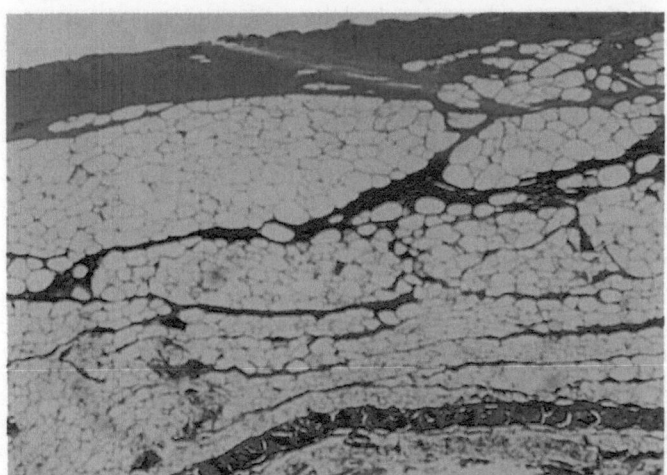

Fig. 7. The depth of the necrosis, colored red in this cross section, reaches just into the subcutaneous fat.

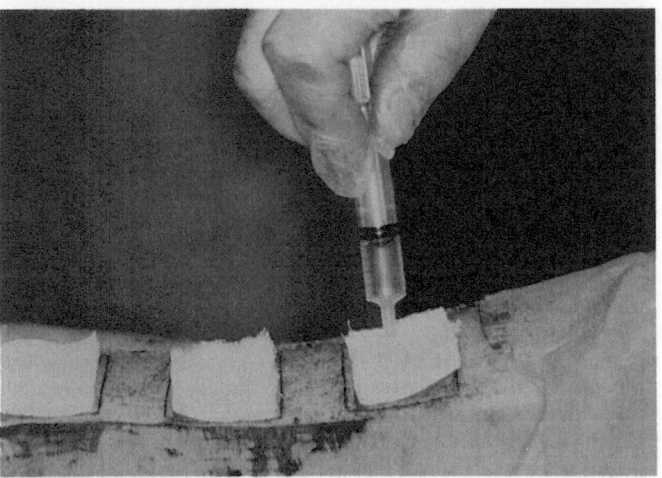

Fig. 8. The remaining wound bed, consisting of a small layer of dermal tissue above the subcutaneous fat, is made necrotic by using an acid.

should realize that removal of necrotic tissue during treatment does not instantly reveal granulation tissue, but it allows for the formation of granulation tissue. Once granulation tissue has been formed near the margin of an ulcer, it will be overgrown with epithelium. As a result, the wound size will be reduced. This means that the relative amount of granulation tissue first increases, but then diminishes. Therefore, the best method for evaluating débridement is to measure the surface covered with necrotic tissue in square millimeters. During the first days of treatment the total wound size may increase as a result of the moisturizing effect of most débriding products.

The good correlation to the visual estimations of an experienced observer may suggest that computer measurements are not necessary. This is not the case, as we have found differences of up to 25% between two observers (unpublished results), and up to 17% when we asked the same observers unexpectedly to evaluate the same ulcer 6 months later. The computer measurements were reproducible; deviations of less than 0.2% were observed, caused by slightly different wound tracings. The system can be used for observer-blind or double-blind clinical studies, multicenter if necessary.

The flexibility of the software makes it suitable for other purposes, like measuring epithelialization in a wound, evaluating laser treatment of pigmented lesions, calculating the percentage of skin covered with psoriasis plaques, and measuring repigmentation in vitiligo spots (Fig. 5) or monoclonal stained cells in histological sections [21]. In conclusion, we recommend that all wound-care products which are said to be suitable for wound cleaning be evaluated with an observer-blind and quantitative system as described above.

References

1. Haury B, Rodeheaver G, Vensko J (1978) Débridement: an essential component of traumatic wound care. Am J Surg 135:238–242
2. Westerhof W, Mekkes JR (1990) Krill and other enzymes in enzymatic wound débridement. In: Wadstrom T, Eliasson I, Holder I, Ljungh A (eds) Pathogenesis of wound and biomaterial-associated infections. Springer, Berlin Heidelberg London New York, pp 180–188
3. Ågren MS, Taplin CJ, Woessner JF jr, Eaglstein WH, Mertz PM (1992) Collagenase in wound healing: effect of wound age and type. J Invest. Dermatol 99:709–714
4. Grøndahl-Hansen J, Lund LR, Ralfkiær E, Ottevanger V, Danø K (1988) Urokinase and tissue-type plasminogen activators in keratinocytes during wound reepithelialization. J Invest Dermatol 90:790–795
5. Chen WYJ, Rogers AA, Lydon MJ (1992) Characterization of biologic properties of wound fluid collected during early stages of wound healing. J Invest Dermatol 99:559–564

6. Tryggvason K, Höyhtyä M, Salo T (1987) Proteolytic degradation of extracellular matrix in tumor invasion. Biochim Biophys Acta 907: 191–217
7. Masure S, Opdenakker G (1989) Cytokine-mediated proteolysis in tissue remodelling. Experienta 45:542–549
8. Matrisian LM (1990) Metalloproteinases and their inhibitors in matrix remodelling. Trends Genet 6:121–125
9. Westerhof W, van Ginkel CJW, Cohen EB, Mekkes JR (1990) Prospective randomized study comparing the débriding effect of krill enzymes and a non-enzymatic treatment in venous leg ulcers. Dermatologica 181:293–297
10. Eriksson G, Eklund AE, Torlegard K, Dauphin E (1979) Evaluation of leg ulcer treatment with stereophotogrammetry. Br J Dermatol 101: 123–131
11. Covington JS, Griffin JW, Mendius RK (1989) Measurement of pressure ulcer volume using dental impression materials: suggestion from the field. Phys Ther 69:690–694
12. Pories WJ, Schaer EW, Jordan DR, Chase J, Parkinson G, Whittaker R, Strain WH, Rob C (1966) The measurement of wound healing. Surg 59: 821–824
13. Smith DJ, Bhat S, Bulgrin JP (1992) Video image analysis of wound repair. Wounds 4:6–15
14. Berg W, Traneroth C, Gunnarson A, Lossing C (1990) A method for measuring pressure sores. Lancet 335:1445–1446
15. Rippon MG, Springett K (1991) Wound healing: validation and application of C-scan ultrasound in human and porcine skin wounds. 1st European Tissue Repair Society Meeting, Oxford, p 96
16. Zahouani H, Assoul M, Janod P, Mignot J (1992) Theoretical and experimental study of wound healing: application to leg ulcers. Med Biol Eng Comput 30:234–239
17. Plassmann P, Jones BF (1992) Measuring leg ulcers by color-coded structured light. J Wound Care 1:35–38
18. Stotts NA (1990) Seeing red, yellow and black. The three-color concept of wound care. Nursing 20:59–61
19. Van Riet Paap E, Mekkes JR, Estevez O, Westerhof W (1991) A new color video image analysis system for the objective assessment of wound healing in secondary healing ulcers. Wounds 3:47
20. Engström N, Hansson F, Hellgren L, Johansson T, Nordin B, Vincent J, Wahlberg A (1990) Computerized wound image analysis. In: Wadstrom T, Eliasson I, Holder I, Ljungh A (eds) Pathogenesis of wound and biomaterial-associated infections. Springer, Berlin Heidelberg London New York, pp 189–192
21. Perednia D (1991) What dermatologists should know about digital imaging. J Am Acad Dermatol 25:89–108

Interview

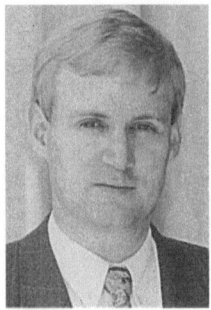

What are the preconditions for modern wound healing studies in your eyes?

Mekkes: To perform clinical research on wound-care products, quantitative and objective methods for the evaluation of wound repair are essential. Usually, the reduction in wound size during treatment is measured.

Why did you develop the new digital image analysis system?

Mekkes: For wound-care products which pretend to débride a wound, objective evaluation of the shift from black/yellow necrosis to red granulation tissue is essential. This is the main reason why we developed the DIA.

How does DIA work?

Mekkes: It uses a video image of an ulcer obtained by positioning a video camera and a light source, both mounted with polaroid filters, in a standardized way in relation to the wound. All variables such as height, distance, angle, light, and diaphragm are recorded. The computer software was specially written by the department of Medical Physics of the Academic Medical Center in Amsterdam. This allows an objective evaluation of the débriding capacity of wound-care products.

Types of Enzymes on the Market

W. Vanscheidt and J. M. Weiss

Summary

Only a few preparations with proteolytic enzymes are commercially available. One is a combination of streptokinase and streptodornase. Streptokinase, an enzyme activator produced by streptococci, is an indirectly acting enzyme and works by transformation of plasminogen to plasmin. Therefore, it can function only in the presence of plasminogen in the wound fluid. Streptodornase is a desoxyribonuclease from streptococci. It degrades nucleic acids to purines and pyrimidines and thereby liquifies the viscous wound exudate. Fibrinolysin, a plasmin from bovine plasma, is combined with a desoxyribonuclease from bovine pancreas and converts fibrin to comparatively large cleavage products.

Trypsin is a proteolytic enzyme of the bovine pancreas. It hydrolyzes ether and peptide bonds and breaks down denatured proteins, but not collagen and elastin. Bromelain is an enzymatic complex of the pineapple. It inhibits platelet aggregation and has fibrinolytic activity. Collagenases from *Clostridium histolyticum* recognize amino acid sequences with great specifity. Sutilain is a proteolytic enzyme from *Bacillus subtilis* and hydrolyzes proteins and is active against fibrin. Krill enzymes from *Euphasia superba* are a combination of endo- and exopeptidases and the most recent development. In contradiction to the clinical importance of proteolytic enzymes, published clinical studies are often outmoded or of inferior quality.

Introduction

There is, worldwide, a high incidence of chronic wounds which require topical treatment. Research in the field of local

Department of Dermatology, University of Freiburg, FRG

enzymatic wound treatment has been neglected until very recently. Therefore, it is not surprising that only a few preparations are commercially available. The aim of this article is to review what is known about the chemical composition, pharmacodynamics, and clinical efficacy of the currently commercially available proteolytic enzymes for wound treatment. Exopeptidases hydrolyze the amino or the carboxy terminal protein, while endopeptidases degrade peptide bonds within the protein molecule.

Streptokinase and Streptodornase

Streptokinase is an enzyme activator from *Streptococcus hemolyticus Lancefield.* Its molecular weight is 47 000. This enzyme has a sedimentation constant of 3.0. Its activity is restricted to a pH between 7.3 and 7.6.

Streptokinase forms a complex with human plasminogen which leads to a change of the conformation of the plasminogen molecule. Hereby, the active center of the molecule is freed. This streptokinase-plasminogen complex is rapidly changed to a streptokinase-plasmin complex. The latter activates plasminogen as well. This mechanism explains why the fibrinolytic activity initially increases with the dosage of streptokinase, and then decreases when there are no more plasminogen molecules available in the wound fluid. Its preferential cleavage points are arginine-valine bonds.

Streptokinase acts indirectly by conversion of plasminogen to plasmin and indirectly enhances degradation of fibrin. Plasmin in turn cleaves fibrin, fibrinogen, factor V, and factor VIII into polypeptides and amino acids.

The wound cleansing efficacy of streptokinase is probably due to the cleavage of fibrin, since the fibrin network on the wound prevents the elimination of necrotic tissue by granulocytes and macrophages.

The efficacy of streptokinase is limited to the presence of plasminogen. Therefore, the topical use of streptokinase is reasonable only if sufficient plasminogen-containing wound exudate is present.

Removal of fibrin implies the risk of inducing bleeding. Therefore, streptokinase is contraindicated on fresh wounds. The risk of sensibilization to streptokinase, which prevents later systemic thrombolysis, is theoretically possible but in fact extremely rare [4, 5, 10, 18, 20].

Streptodornase is another enzyme of *Streptococcus hemolyticus* of the Lancefield group. This deoxyribonuclease is active on a broad pH range with a maximum of 7.5. By degradation of nucleic acids to purines (adenine, guanine) and pyrimidines (cytosine, thymidine), the viscous wound exudate is liquified. This enzyme works by an endonucleolytic cleavage to 3,-phosphodinucleotide and 3,-phosphodinucleotide end-products in double-stranded DNA. Streptodornase attacks no vital structures within a wound. The resorption of cleaved purines and pyrimidines can cause fever, chills, and leukocytosis. Treatment for longer than 2–3 weeks may be associated with decreasing débriding activity. A combination of streptokinase/streptodornase is commercially available.

The débriding activity of a streptokinase/streptodornase preparation was evaluated on rat skin and showed about 10% of the débriding capacity of a yet experimental débriding enzymatic preparation (krill) [3, 9].

Clinical Efficacy

The cleansing effect of streptokinase in combination with streptodornase was evaluated in a study of 40 patients with venous or arterial leg ulcers. The débriding activity was high concerning pus and débris. The combination was unable to remove deep necrosis in arterial leg ulcers, however. The bacterial contamination of the leg ulcers was reduced, probably due to the removal of necrotic tissue [10]. In another randomized study streptokinase in combination with streptodornase proved to be more effective than topical saline solution [5].

Skog [30] performed a study on 24 patients with chronic venous arterial leg ulcers or infected leg ulcers. The clinical results were evaluated by a score for removal of necrosis and induction of granulation. The leg ulcer size was measured dur-

Table 1. Clinical studies with streptokinase/streptodornase.

Type of study	Inclusion	Number	Control	Results	Reference
Single-blind	Leg ulcers	31	Saline	>> Saline	[5]
Open	ENT wounds	30	None	+ +	[34]
Open	Surgical wounds	24	None	+ +	[20]
Open	Surgical wounds	34	None	+ +	[18]
Open	Leg ulcers	24	None	+ +	[30]

ing the treatment. In arterial leg ulcers there was no effect on gangrene. Four of them healed during treatment. Only one of seven venous leg ulcers healed during the treatment, while débridement of necrosis and induction of granulation were judged to be positive in most of the cases.

Remarkable was the effect on the necrosis of infected leg ulcers. In all cases it was possible to remove the necrotic tissue. The author observed that the main effect of the local treatment occurred within 2–3 weeks. Longer treatment periods seem to be less promising.

Other publications report mainly clinical experience. Lang [18] treated 34 patients with pressure sores, infected wounds, osteomyelitis, and fistulas with streptokinase in combination with streptodornase. Healthy granulation tissue developed generally within a week, with no effect on the healthy tissue. Wound infection was reduced.

Überfeldt [34] treated necrotic purulent wounds in the ENT field and was rapidly able to obtain fresh granulation tissue. No side effects were observed.

Secondary healing of wounds of 24 patients was achieved with this combination, as reported by Lenz and Hoffmann [20]. In all cases formation of fresh granulation tissue was found, and no allergic side effects were observed.

Fibrinolysin and Deoxyribonuclease

Fibrinolysin is a plasmin produced from bovine plasma, where it is present as an inactive precursor. This precursor is extracted and activated by chloroform. It is not soluble in water and has an isoelectric point of 5.5. Dried fibrinolysin is stable; once dissolved, its enzymatic activity is lost within 6–8 h. Fibrinolysin converts fibrin to comparatively large cleavage products and inactivates fibrinogen and coagulation factors I, V, and VII and locally dilates the blood vessels in the wound. It preferentially cleaves lysine-arginine bonds. In contrast to streptokinase, it is directly active and therefore not dependent on the presence of plasminogen in the wound exudate. By the cleavage of fibrin and dissolution of coagula, necrotic tissue becomes accessible for débridement by wound macrophages. The large split products are not systemically resorbed but rather drained with the wound exudate.

Deoxyribonuclease is a DNase which originates from bovine pancreas. It cleaves nuclear substances with a preference for double-stranded DNA and liquefies the exudate by decreasing its viscosity. It works by endonucleolytic cleavage of 5,phosphodinucleotide and 5-phospho-oligonucleotide end-products. Its molecular weight is 60000; its isoelectric point lies between pH 4.7 and 5.0. A diluted watery solution remains stable within a wide range of pH at a temperature of 5°C. With an increase of temperature the activity of this enzyme rapidly decreases. The activity is regained after cooling. Since pus consists largely of nucleoproteins and fibrinous components, a combination with fibrinolysin seems entirely appropriate. A combination of fibrinolysin/deoxyribonuclease is commercially available [4, 26, 31, 35].

Clinical Efficacy

The débriding activity of fibrinolysin was evaluated on rat skin and showed about 10% of the débriding capacity of a yet experimental débriding enzymatic preparation (krill) [3].

In a clinical trial of 42 patients with secondary healing wounds a combination of fibrinolysin/deoxyribonuclease was evaluated for its therapeutic value concerning clinical efficacy and tolerability. The therapeutic success was estimated to be good. The solution seemed to be more effective than the ointment [26].

In a study of 30 patients with second- and third-degree burn wounds fibrinolysin/deoxyribonuclease proved to be superior to silver nitrate [24].

In a randomized single-blind study 44 patients with wound healing disorders were treated with either fibrinolysin/deoxyribonuclease (group 1) or streptokinase/streptodornase (group 2). Group 1 seemed to be slightly superior to group 2 [31].

Table 2. Clinical studies of fibrinolysin deoxyribonuclease

Type of study	Inclusion	Number	Control	Results	Reference
Open	Surgical wounds	42	None	+ +	[26]
Open	Burn wounds	30	Silver nitrate	F >> Silver nitrate	[24]
Single-blind	Surgical wounds	44	ST/SD	F >> ST/SD	[31]
Open	Surgical wounds	30	None	+ +	[16]
Open	Leg ulcers	34	Saline	F >> Saline	[35]

Thirty patients with secondary healing wounds were treated with fibrinolysin/deoxyribonuclease, and the clinical results were reported to be satisfying [16]. In another study, 25 patients were treated with fibrinolysin/deoxyribonuclease solution. In 15 cases the previously therapy-resistant wounds healed completely. Nine patients were dismissed from hospital before wound healing was completed, but their wounds had started to heal. There was only one therapy failure [13]. In a multicenter study of 258 patients three topical enzyme preparations were compared: fibrinolysin/deoxyribonuclease, clostridiopeptidase with chloramphenicol, and trypsin with framycetin sulfate. Concerning the clinical efficacy, no significant differences were observed between the three preparations. The frequency of side effects was higher, however, in the two antibiotic-containing preparations, due mainly to allergic reactions [4].

In a controlled, randomized, double-blind study of 34 chronic leg ulcer patients, 37 leg ulcers were treated with either fibri-

Fig. 1. Surgical Débridement of a venous leg ulcer.

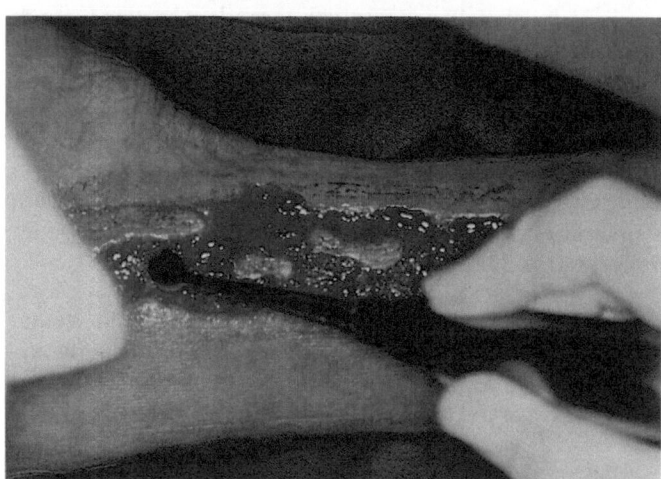

Fig. 2. Diagram of Fibrinolysin.

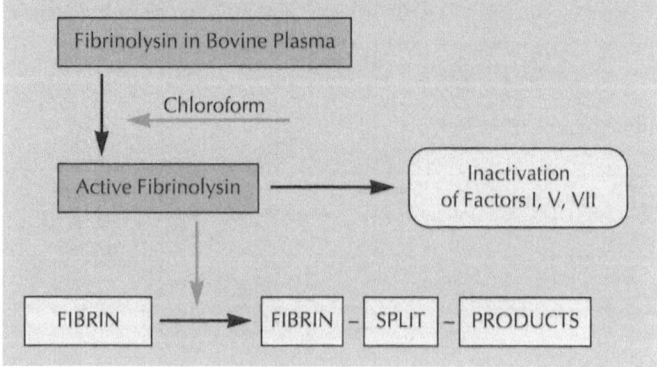

nolysin/deoxyribonuclease (verum) or saline solution (placebo). Verum was significantly more effective concerning cleansing of the wounds and increasing granulation than placebo in venous leg ulcer patients. This difference was not significant if combined leg ulcers were treated [35].

Trypsin

Trypsin is a crystalline proteolytic enzyme of the bovine pancreas. It hydrolyzes ether and peptide bonds consisting mainly of amino acids, where the majority of amino acids are lysine or arginine. Trypsin breaks down denatured proteins, but not collagen and elastin. It liquefies blood coagula and wound scabs. Its temperature optimum corresponds to the body temperature.

Clinical Efficacy

The débriding activity of trypsin was evaluated on rat skin and showed about 50% of the débriding capacity of a yet experimental débriding enzymatic preparation (krill) [3].

Forty patients with venous leg ulcers or arterial leg ulcers were treated either with streptokinase/streptodornase or with stabilized trypsin. Both preparations showed a total or subtotal cleansing effect on necrotic tissue within the wound and enhanced granulation tissue formation. Concerning pus and necrosis, streptokinase/streptodornase proved to be superior. No preparation was able to remove deep necrosis in arterial ulcers, however. Both treatments led to a reduction of bacterial contamination of the ulcers, probably due to elimination of necrotic material [10].

In a study of 328 patients, 110 were treated with trypsin inactivated on cellulose, 148 with unmodified trypsin, and 70 with

Type of study	Inclusion	Number	Control	Results	Reference
Table 3. Clinical studies of trypsin					
Randomized	Leg ulcers	40	ST/SD	ST/SD >> trypsin	[10]
Open	Surgical wounds	110	Antiseptics	Trypsin >> antiseptics	[37]
Open	Surgical wounds	128	Collocoyl	+ +	[33]

antiseptics. This comparative study gave evidence that inactivated trypsin might have slight advantages [7].
In another study the efficacy of cellulose-inactivated trypsin and collagenase were evaluated. Both preparations accelerated the cleaning of wounds with difficult access, reduced infections, and positively influenced the wound healing process [33].

In several countries side effects such as itching or pain have led to withdrawal of trypsin-based preparations from the market.

Fig. 3. Diagram of Trypsin.

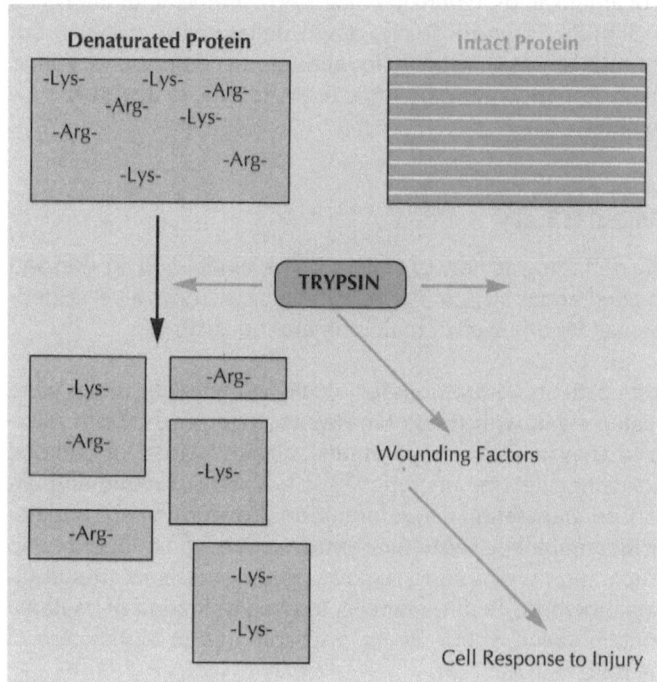

Bromelain

Bromelain is an enzymatic complex of the pineapple. Christopher Columbus reported that warriors of the Caribbean islands treated wounds with pineapple juice. Even though the exact chemical structure of all active components of bromelain has not yet been identified, this substance has interesting pharmacological effects: [12]

- Interference with the growth of tumor cells
- Inhibition of platelet aggregation
- Fibrinolytic activity
- Antiinflammatory effects
- Wound cleansing

Its effects are probably due to an interference with the arachidonic acid metabolism in the wound. Bromelain was shown to successfully débride experimental burns in pigs without damaging unburned skin [14].

Clinical Efficacy

The necrolytic activity of bromelain was investigated in rats with third-degree burn wounds. With use of a 35% concentration a total and selective cleansing of the wounds was observed. Histologically, no effect on the neighboring tissue was seen. Combination with PVP iodine completely inhibits this enzyme, while sulfadiazine and gentamicin have no detrimental effect [17].

In another study, the efficacy of bromelain in frostbite was evaluated. Third-degree cold wounds were experimentally induced on pig skin with liquid nitrogen. Thereafter, the wounds were topically treated with bromelain. Bromelain had no significant effect. It was concluded that the lack of coagulated proteins inactivates bromelain too rapidly [1].

Table 4. Experimental studies with bromelain.

Type of study	Inclusion	Number	Control	Results	Reference
Experimental, on rat skin	Burn wounds	30	None	High efficacy	[17]
Experimental, on pig skin	Frostbite	15	None	Slight efficacy	[1]

Collagenase

Collagenases recognize with great specificity the amino acid sequence at which they attack, within the helical regions of native collagen. Collagen is degraded to small fragments. It preferentially cleaves glycine in the sequence x-proline-y-glycine-proline-z. Presumably, these are sterically weak points in the triple-helix structure of the collagen molecule.

Collagenases are commercially available in combination with chloramphenicol or as a monoproduct. The main product is derived from *Clostridium histolyticum.* Another collagenase from *Achromobacter iophagus* has recently been investigated as well.

Clinical Efficacy

After intradermal injections of collagenase, hyaluronidase, and a combination of both, the last proved to be most effective concerning degradation of connective matrix, followed by collagenase. Hyaluronidase had only minimal effects [7].

ACR-59 is a collagenase from *Achromobacter iophagus*. After thermal injury to the backs of male Wister rats, burned and healthy skin was immediately excised and treated with ACR-59 (HCl buffered, pH = 7.2, 37°C). The degradation of the skin specimen was measured by hydroxyproline. At concentrations of about 0.03 nkat/ml ACR-59, this was achieved in a dose-dependent manner. For healthy skin, however, concentrations of 30 nkat/ml were required.

Fibroblasts from fetal rat skin were cultivated in Dulbecco's modified Eagles medium. At concentrations of 3.125 nkat/ml the cell proliferation was increased by ACR-59; it was inhibited at concentrations of > 25 nkat/ml.

Percutaneous absorption of ACR-59 ointment was investigated on the backs of rats and rabbits. The ointment was topically applied with an occlusive dressing. At regular intervals the ACR-59 concentrations were determined by enzyme immunoassay (EIA) and enzymatic activity. On healthy skin no ACR-59 was measured after treatment with 50 μkat/g/kg for rats and 2 μkat/g/kg for rabbits. Percutaneous absorption was demonstrated after topical application on "stripped" skin, while on burn wounds and other open wounds this was somehow inhibited. For further data on collagenases, see Hatz et al., this volume.

Table 5. Clinical studies of collagenases (*Ulc. dermat.* ulcerative dermatitis, + + positive, F combination of fibrinolysin/deoxyribonuclease, *ST/SD* combination of streptokinase/streptodornase, *Collag.* collagenase).

Type of study	Inclusion	Number	Control	Results	Reference
Open	Ulc. dermat.	20	None	+ +	[8]
Open	Leg ulcers	95	None	+ +	[21]
Open	Suppurative wounds	239	None	+ +	[15]
Open	Leg ulcers	258	F ST/SD	n.s.	[5]
Open	Leg ulcers	20	None	+ +	[19]
Double-blind	Leg ulcers	30	Placebo	Collag. >> Placebo	[23]

Clinical Studies

A topical combination of collagenases and chloramphenicol induced a rapid cleansing of wounds due to ulcerative dermatitis [8]. Ninety-five patients with chronic ulcers were treated with this combination in another study. In all cases the results proved to be satisfying [21]. In a Russian study, 239 patients with suppurative skin lesions were treated with a collagenase preparation. The removal of necrotic tissue was enhanced [15]. Lazzari [19] reported positive clinical results with collagenases in a clinical trial on 20 leg-ulcer patients. Palmieri [23] treated 30 patients in a double-blind study and showed that collagenase was superior to placebo.

Sutilain

Sutilain is a proteolytic enzyme from *Bacillus subtilis,* discovered in 1960. It hydrolyzes proteins and digests necrotic tissue and denatured collagen. In vitro, sutilain is active against fibrin and somewhat less against proteins, hemoglobin, and collagen [27]. Its pH optimum lies between 6 and 6.8 [12].

Clinical Efficacy

Good results were reported after treatment of burns with sutilain [27]. Major side effects were a burning sensation in the wound and mild inflammation of the healthy neighboring skin. Treatment is contraindicated for ulcers communicating with major body cavities or those containing exposed nerves, and for neoplastic ulcers [12]. Systemic allergic reactions have not been reported; antibody formation can occur due to absorption of the enzyme [27].

Krill Enzymes

First experimental and clinical studies with the new krill enzyme system of endo- and exopeptidases have been reported. The predominant activity is caused by the endopeptidases, exo-

Table 6. Clinical studies of krill enzymes					
Type of study	Inclusion	Number	Control	Results	Reference
Randomized	Leg ulcers	31	Non-enzymatic	Krill >> non-enzymatic	[36]

Fig. 4. Diagram of Krill Enzymes.

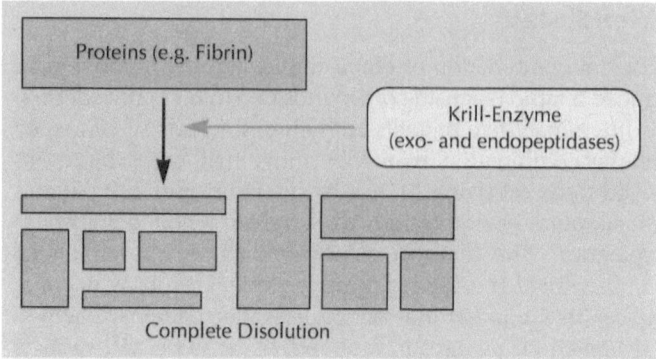

peptidases being cooperative enzymes. Their pH optimum is alkaline, and they require much less activation energy than mammalian enzymes [9]. Published and ongoing studies in several European countries seem to support observations that the krill enzymes are very potent débriders.

Conclusion

Undoubtedly, enzymatic wound débriders are essential for the treatment of patients with chronic wounds and burns. Due to the high incidence of wounds world wide, further experimental and clinical research in this field is urgently recommended.

References

1. Ahle NW (1987) Enzymatic frostbite eschar débridement by bromelain. Ann Emerg Med. Sep; 16(9):1063–1065
2. Anheller JE, Hellgren L, Karlstam B, Vincent J (1989) Biochemical and biological profile of a new enzyme preparation from antarctic krill (E. superba) suitable for débridement of ulcerative lesions. Arch Dermatol Res 281, No. 2, pp 105–110
3. Campbell D, Hellgren L, Karlstam B, Vincent J (1987) Débriding ability of a novel multi-enzym preparation isolatet from antarctic krill (Euphausia superba). Experientia 43, No 5, pp 578–579
4. Fischer H, Gilliet F, Hornemann M, Leyh F, Lindemayr H, Stegmann W, Welke S (1984) Enzymatische Wundreinigung beim venosen Ulcus cruris. Bericht über eine multizentrische klinische Vergleichsstudie mit verschiedenen Enzympräparaten. Fortschr Med 102:281–283
5. Forsling E (1988) Comparison of saline and streptokinase-streptodornase in the treatment of leg ulcers. Eur J Clin Pharmacol 33:637–638
6. Friedman (1986) Degradation of porcine dermal connective tissue by collagenase and hyaluronidas. Br. J Dermatol 115:403–408
7. Gostishchev VK, Tolstykh PI, Khanin AG, Vasilkova ZF, Iusupov KA (1985) Trypsin, immobilized on a textile cellulose matrix, in the treatment of suppurative wounds of soft tissues (in Russian). Vestn Khir 134:68–71

8. Graifemberghi S (1984) Use of collagenase and nonspecific proteases in the treatment of necrotic ulcerative dermatitis. Clin Ter 110:359–362
9. Hellgren L, Mohr V, Vincent J (1986) Proteases of Antarctic krill – a new system for effective enzymatic débridement of necrotic ulcerations. Experientia 42:403–404
10. Hellgren L (1983) Cleansing properties of stabilized trypsin and streptokinase-streptodornase in necrotic leg ulcers. Eur J Clin Pharmacol 24:623–628
11. Hellgren L, Vincent J (1977) Degradation and liquefaction effect of streptokinase-streptodornase and stabilyzed trypsin on necrosis, crusts of fibrinoid, purulent exudate and clotted blood from leg ulcers. J Int Med Res 5:334–338
12. Hellgren L, Vincent J (1993) personal communication
13. Herzberg E (1989) Behandlung problematischer septischer Wunden. Zeitschrift für Allgemeinmedizin 1303–1304
14. Houck J (1983) Isolation of an effective débriding agent from the stems of pineapple plants. Int J Tissue React 5:125–134
15. Kharitonov IuK, Berchenko GN, Berchenko VV, Aboiants RK (1986) Treatment of suppurative wounds of soft tissues with colocyl and its combination with proteolytic enzymes (in russian) Vestn Khir 137:63–66
16. Kroath F (1984) Erfahrungen mit der enzymatischen Wundreinigung. Therapiewoche 34:2609–2612
17. Klaue P, Aman G, Romen W (1979) Chemical débridement of the burn eschar in rats with bromelain combined with topical antimicrobial agents. Eur Sur Res 11:353–359
18. Lang HD (1981) Wirksamkeit und Verträglichkeit von Varidase bei Ulzerationen, sekundärer Wundheilung und Osteomyelitiden. Therapiewoche 31:6652–6656
19. Lazzari G (1990) Collagenase for the treatment of torpide ulcerative lesions of the legs. Ital Dermatol Venereol 125:37–42
20. Lenz J, Hoffmann W (1980) Erfahrungen mit Varidase-Gel bei sekundär verheilenden Weichteildefekten. Klinikarzt 9:210–212
21. Mariotti U, Bellomo F (1984) The use of collagenase-clostridiopeptidase combined with chloramphenicol in orthopaedics and traumatology. Ital J Orthop Traumatol 10:405–410
22. Mekkes JR, Westerhof W (1990) Proteolytic débridement of necrotic wounds using krill enzymes in a pig model. J Invest Dermatol 95:480–485
23. Palmieri R (1993) personal communication
24. Roman-Calderon J (1982) Treatment of second and third degree burns: Comparison of effects of proteolytic enzyme combination and silver nitrate. Curr Ther Res 32:305–311
25. Reames MK, Christensen C, Luce EA (1988) The use of maggots in wound débridement. Ann Plast Surg 21:388–391
26. Schwarz N (1981) Erfahrungen bei der Wundreinigung mit der Enzymkombination Fibrinolysin/Desoxyribonuklease. Fortschr Med 25:978–980
27. Shakespeare PG (1979) The activity of the enzymatic débridement agent travase towards a variety of protein substrates. Burn 6:15–20
28. Sherry S, Goeller J (1950) The extent of enzymatic degradation of DNA in purulent exudates by streptodornase. Clin Invest 29:1588–1594
30. Skog F (1984) Behandlung schwer heilbarer Beinulcera mit Streptokinase-Streptodornase-Lösung. Opuscula medica 34

31. Stüwe U (1983) Enzymatische Wundreinigung – Vergleich zweier handelsüblicher Medikamente. Fortschr Med 41:1883–1888

32. Taussig SJ, Batkin S (1988) Bromelain, the enzyme complex of pineapple (ananas comosus) and its clinical application. An update. J Ethnopharmacol 22:191–203

33. Tostykh PI, Titov AI, Vartanian ZhS, Derbenev VA, Danilova TM, Dadashev AI (1990) Characteristics of wound process after high-energy laser débridement and enzyme treatment (in russian). Khirurgiia 6:12–16

34. Ueberfeldt N (1980) Erfahrungen mit Streptokinase-Streptodornase (Varidase) in der HNO-Heilkunde. Med Klin 14: 524–525

35. Westerhof W, Jansen FC, de Wit FS, Cormane RH (1987) Controlled double-blind trial of fibrinolysin-desoxyribonuclease (Elase) solution in patients with chronic leg ulcers who are treated before autologous skin grafting. J Am Acad Dermatol 17:32–39

36. Westerhof W, van Ginkel GJ, Cohen EB, Mekkes JR (1990) Prospective randomized study comparing the débriding effect of krill enzymes and a non-enzymatic treatment in venous leg ulcers. Dermatologica 181: 293–297

Interview

What is your impression about research on the treatment of chronic wounds?

Vanscheidt: Research in this field has been surprisingly neglected in the past. The increase of knowledge about wound healing in general is very impressive, but the quantity and quality of research on treatment is quite deficient.

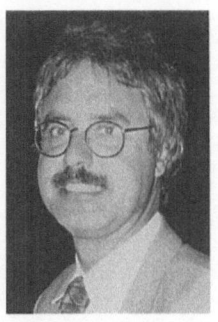

What is missing in this area of research?

Vanscheidt: Very few clinical studies have been performed on the effectiveness of the currently available proteolytic enzymes. In particular, double-blind multicenter studies are rare. Even rarer are studies which use objective measurements of the débriding capacity of the preparations.

What is the most effective preparation on the market?

Vanscheidt: Due to the lack of studies with the aforementioned quality it is still too early to prove that one enzyme is superior to the other. The twofold concentration of collagenase without an antibiotic is promising. I personally have high hopes for this new preparation which, however, need verification by clinical studies on a high scientific level.

The Role of Collagenase in Wound Healing

R. A. Hatz, N. C. S. von Jan, and F. W. Schildberg

Summary

Specific collagenases possess the unique capability of degrading native collagen otherwise resistant to breakdown by all other proteases. In wound healing mesenchymal cells release collagenase into the extracellular matrix and phagocytic cells lyse collagen, either on their surface or intracellularly. Collagenase production is stimulated by interleukin-1, the platelet-derived growth factor (PDGF), and others. Several factors terminate collagenase activity; the most potent is alpha-2-macroglobulin. The best characterized bacterial collagenase is produced by *Clostridium histolyticum*. In contrast to a variety of other clinically tested enzymes, collagenases are the only proteases which can specifically hydrolyze native collagen. Wound healing can be accelerated by enhancement of macrophage chemotaxis due to collagen-derived peptides generated by bacterial collagenase. An increase in macrophage numbers will lead to enhanced cytokine secretion in wounds. In third-degree burn wounds, the event of hypertrophic scarring and scar contracture was markedly reduced in collagenase-treated wounds. Further studies are needed to clarify these effects of collagenase.

Introduction

Wound healing is the complex response to tissue injury controlled by local and migrated cells. Our knowledge of the underlying biochemical features is constantly being enriched by tremendous advances in cellular and molecular biology. Therefore, it is important to coordinate and organize new insights and to focus in particular on the role of the degrading enzyme collagenase, ubiquitous in healing wounds. Specific collagenases possess the unique capability of degrading na-

Department of Surgery, Klinikum Grosshadern, Ludwig-Maximilians-University, Munich, Germany

Table 1. Collagenase activity increased/decreased with selected conditions.

Healing wounds	↑
Post-burn granulation tissue	↑
Keloids	↓
Hypertrophic scar	↑
Bone resorption	↑
Anastomotic insufficiency of the bowel	↑
Periodontitis	↑
Diabetic rats	↑
Rheumatoid arthritis	↑

tive collagen, which is resistant to breakdown by other known tissue proteases [1]. Reports suggest that degradation products of collagen released after cleavage by collagenase may in turn effect the migration and activity of important inflammatory cells such as wound macrophages, and therefore at a very early stage in wound repair substantially influence the healing process [2–4]. Abnormal collagen deposition as a result of alterations in collagenolysis may be seen in various pathologic conditions, such as hypertrophic scars and keloids [5]. Excessively high collagenase activity is found in rheumatoid arthritis, local tumor invasion, excessive bone resorption following bone injury, anastomotic insufficiency following bowel surgery, and post-burn granulation tissue [6–11] (Table 1). Selective therapeutic enhancement or blockage of the collagenolytic system may therefore prove to be a valuable tool in treatment or prevention of these conditions.

Mammilian Collagenases

Mammilian collagenase is an endoprotease (i. e., proteinase) which cleaves collagen molecules at its triple-helical main structure at neutral physiologic pH and temperature. There is one susceptible sequence which predetermines decomposition, placed at two thirds of the molecule (Fig. 2). The specificity with which mammilian collagenases cleave their substrate at a definite site is truly remarkable: The target amino acid sequence is gly-ile in collagen type I, which appears three times in the alpha-1- chain, and gly-leu in collagen type III, appearing 18 times in the alpha-1 chain. The cleavage of collagen type I always takes place between residues 775 and 776 of the alpha-1 chain. This seems to be a weak point in the triple-helical structure, resulting in typical lengths of cleaved fibrils,

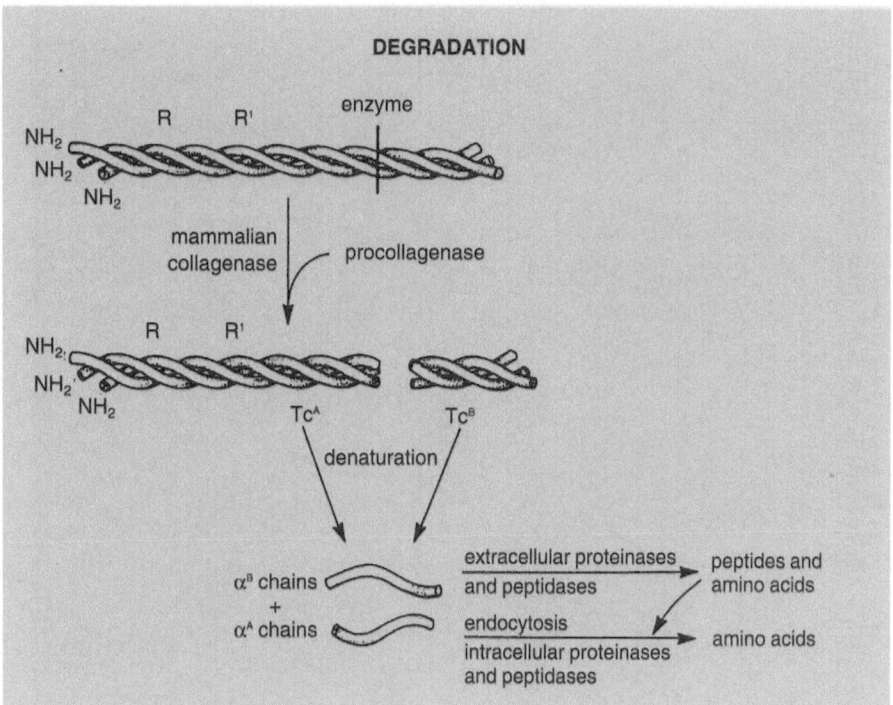

DEGRADATION

enzyme

R   R'

NH₂
NH₂
NH₂

mammalian collagenase   procollagenase

R   R'

NH₂
NH₂
NH₂

Tcᴬ   Tcᴮ

denaturation

αᴮ chains
+
αᴬ chains

extracellular proteinases and peptidases → peptides and amino acids

endocytosis
intracellular proteinases and peptidases → amino acids

¾ and ¼ of the helix. Collagen types II and III have comparable results after cleavage. Consequently, chains appear to be parted into long N-terminal and short C-terminal fractions. This result proves cleavage by a real collagenase.

Fig. 1. Scheme showing cleavage of collagen by mammalian collagenase.

Localization

Only two biochemically distinct interstitial collagenases have been described to date: the human neutrophil collagenase (HNC) [12] and the human fibroblast collagenase (HFC) [13]. These are the best characterized. They are capable of degrading interstitial types I–III collagens. Two type-IV collagenases (= gelatinases) in 72- and 92-kDa forms have been described. However, their biological function has not yet been clearly defined. They degrade type-V, -VII and -X collagens and gelatin. As to the ubiquitous presence of connective tissue, the two interstitial collagenase types HNC and HFC are produced by a number of mesenchymal cells. Collagenase is not an intracellularly stored enzyme, nor is it constantly released. Its synthesis is initiated only on request. This makes collagenase extraction from tissue most difficult. Therefore, knowledge as to the different sites of its production is still incomplete. As a matter of fact, fibroblasts in the upper papillary dermis produce more collagenase than those in epidermal areas. In wound healing

Table 2. Important regulatory peptides in wound healing (*EGF* epidermal growth factor, *TGFα/β* transforming growth factor α/β, *a/bFGF* acidic/basic fibroblast growth factor, *MGF* macrophage growth factor, *MDGF* macrophage derived growth factor, *PDGF* platelet-derived growth factor, *IL-I* interleukin-1, *TNFα* tumor necrosis factor α, *IFNγ* interferon γ).

Peptide	Main source	Biological effect on					Collagenase release	Remarks
		White blood cells	Endothelial cells	Fibroblasts	Keratinocytes	Collagen production		
EGF	present in most body fluids		chemotactic, mitogenic	chemotactic, mitogenic	mitogenic	increased, inhibition	no stimulation	TGFα has mostly the same effects
FGF	aFGF: brain retina, chemotactic? bFGF: brain, retina macrophages		chemotactic, mitogenic	chemotactic, mitogenic		increased	stimulation	bFGF is identical with MGF, MDGF
TGFβ	platelets, macrophages, endoth. cells	chemotactic on neutrophils, monocytes	growth inhibition, mitogenic	chemotactic, inhibitory, and mitogenic	reversible growth inhibition	increased, inhibition of degradation	inhibition upregulation of type IV, stimulation	combination with PDGF potentiates collagen deposition
PDGF	platelets, macrophages, endoth. cells	chemotactic on neutrophils monocytes	no effect, mitogenic on vasc, smooth muscle cells	chemotactic, mitogenic		stimulation of type V formation, parallel decrease of type III in gingival fibroblasts	stimulation	inhibits EGF
IL-I	neutrophils, monocytes, macrophages, endoth. cells, keratinocytes	chemotactic	growth inhibition, activation, mito-genic on smooth muscle cells	mitogenic	chemotactic, mitogenic	stimulation	stimulation	induction of IFNγ, PDGF release
TNFα	monocytes, macrophages, keratinocytes	chemotactic on neutrophils	chemotactic, in vitro: inhibition, in vivo: mitogenic	mitogenic	stimulates TGFα (potent auto-crine growth factor) release	stimulation, inhibition	stimulation	induction of PDGF release; inhibits TGFβ-induced collagen synthesis

two types of collagenase have been detected, one synthesized by epithelial cells, the other by granulation tissue. Large amounts of collagenase have been found in supernatants of synovial cell cultures, derived from patients suffering from primary chronic arthritis. Its production is triggered by interleukin-1, in this case leading to the destruction of collagen-containing structures of the joint. Collagenase activity has been confirmed by examination of the collagen fractions.

Another known location of collagenase production is gingival tissue, as it has been detected near erosions which are found in gingivitis/periodontitis. The characteristic breakdown of connective tissue is initiated by bacterial plaques on teeth triggering mononuclear cells, which in turn release factors activating collagenase.

Most important, however, considerable amounts of tissue breakdown and remodeling take place at the site of classic inflammation. Therefore, it was suspected early on that hematopoietic cells invading these sites are capable of producing collagenase; this was later confirmed: azurophilic granules of granulocytes contain collagenase aside from elastase and chymotrypsin.

Lymphocytes, monocytes, and macrophages produce collagenase and at the same time secrete lymphokines and monokines, triggering collagenase synthesis by fibroblasts (Table 2). There are two known mechanisms of collagenase-mediated breakdown of collagen by neutrophilic granulocytes. Extracellularly, partly cleaved fibrils are taken up by the phagocyte via endocytosis and completely digested by intracellular proteases stored in azurophilic granules. Cleavage also takes place in pocket-like structures on the surface of phagocytes, which largely protect collagenase from serum inactivators. These pockets can be identified in electron-microscopic preparations and have been called "ruffled borders". The importance of the intracellular location of collagenase activity is further underlined by the fact that collagenase secreted into the extracellular matrix is immediately inactivated by serum-derived inhibitory factors.

In conclusion, there are two main cell groups responsible for collagenase-mediated collagen breakdown: de novo synthesizing mesenchymal cells releasing collagenase into extracellular matrix, where it takes effect, and phagocytic cells storing the enzyme in intracellular granula, lysing collagen either on their surface or intracellularly. The interaction of these two types might play a key role in the regulation of rapid tissue breakdown.

Regulation of Synthesis and Activation

How collagenase production is regulated has been studied most intensively in synovial cells of patients with rheumatoid arthritis. By adding peripheral blood monocytes to cell cultures of dendritic cells, collagenase production is triggered in a reciprocal manner. The reason for this was attributed to a 14- to 24-kDa protein produced by monocytes, which was found to be interleukin-1. Several laboratories have stated its responsibility for the induction of fibroblast collagenase synthesis [14, 15]. Baur et al. showed that PDGF stimulates human skin collagenase expression in vitro [16]. Other factors influencing collagenase synthesis are TGF-β1, bFGF, PGE$_2$ (increase), indomethacin (decrease by inhibiting PGE$_2$ synthesis), vitamin A and corticosteroids (decrease), and the Fc-portion of IgG (increase by stimulating macrophages).

What mechanism activates the "sleeping" ubiquitous enzyme? Since the consequences of tissue destruction in case of a control defect may be fatal, it has to be a highly sensitive pathway. In vivo experiments have shown several factors like cathepsin B, plasmin, and callicrein to activate collagenase directly. Unnamed factors have been detected to promote collagenase synthesis in macrophages of the rabbit lung and rat uterus post partum. Also it was found that progesterone indirectly inhibits collagenase secretion by suppressing the activating factor.

In vitro activation can be elicited by a number of reagents reacting with thio- or disulfides and by proteases such as trypsin, plasmin, chymotrypsin, cathepsin B, callicrein, and thermolysin. The exact biochemical process taking place in activation is yet unknown. It is most probably an enzyme-linked inhibitor which is decleaved, or the zymogen is activated by cleavage at some part of the molecule. The activating mechanism in human neutrophilic granulocytes is more defined and might be transferable to other sites: latent collagenase appears to be a mixed disulfide consisting of active collagenase (65.5–67 kDa) and an inhibitor (20–25 kDa). The enzyme is activated by reduction of the disulfide linkage. Interaction with the glutathione redox system provides regulation and continuation of metabolic events. Collagenase can also be activated by conformation change without any measureable molar weight loss/gain (as an effect of chaotropic reagents in vitro and human serum factors, human skin elements, and rat uterus elements in vivo).

The presence of double-charged metallic ions (Ca^{++} and Zn^{++}) is highly important with respect to possible activation, stability, and effectiveness of the enzyme [17]. Macartney et al. showed that PMN leukocyte collagenase requires zinc for activation by various disulfides. This process was reversible by adding EDTA or cysteine. If zinc and EDTA were given in the same amount, the enzyme was active. A higher concentration of zinc (3 × EDTA) had an inhibitory effect on the activation process.

The two structurally distinct collagenases differ in their reactivity towards various collagen types: human fibroblast collagenase (HFC), for example, lyses type I collagen as well as type III, whereas the human neutrophil collagenase (HNC) attacks type I much more quickly than type III. Type II generally seems to be more resistant to collagenolytic influence than the other types. This has to be ascribed to different three-dimensional factors, especially to the amount of fibril cross-linkings. The reason for the considerable speed of collagen degradation in the postpartum uterus might be a relatively small number of cross-links due to its young age. The resulting collagen fractions are denatured at lower temperatures than the native molecule, e.g., type I at 32°C, which results in instability of the triple-helical structure. Subsequently, susceptibility to nonspecific proteases increases and degradation is accelerated.

There are several factors which terminate collagenase activity: the most potent plasma-derived inhibitor is alpha-2-macroglobulin – due to its molecular size, active only when transported out of blood vessels together with other blood components or in case of vessel disruption. Thus, inhibitors of smaller molecular size play a major role, such as a specific beta-1-collagenase inhibitor (40 kDa) and alpha-1-antitrypsin (54 kDa). The latter is known to inhibit collagenases of skin fibroblasts, neutrophilic granulocytes, thrombocytes, and human synovium. Interestingly, it has been found that parts of the procollagen peptide, released into the extracellular matrix during collagen synthesis, act as inhibitors of collagenase, thereby protecting the newly built molecule from inactivation.

Bacterial Collagenases

Bacterial collagenases were discovered long before mammalian ones. They have been used mostly in laboratories, but also as pharmacological agents [18]. The best-characterized bacterial collagenase is produced by *Clostridium histolyticum*, easily available since it is secreted by the bacterium into the culture medium in large quantities. In contrast to mammalian collagenases, bacterial collagenase activity results in small

Table 3. Bacterial collagenase in clinical wound treatment.

– Débridement
  High affinity for all major collagen types (I–V)

– Enhancement of granulation tissue formation
  Increased chemotaxis and activation of wound macrophages
  mediated by products of collagen degradation (peptides)

– Prevention of pathologic scar formation
  Modulation of collagen type I/III ratio

peptides at an approximate size of five amino acids. Some larger residues have also been detected. It was demonstrated that short segments are clipped off sequentially from each end of the molecule. The initial reactions of digestion seem to be of the first order; with increasing amounts of cleaved particles, second-order reactions predominate.

Clostridium histolyticum-derived collagenase cleaves all five collagen types at nearly the same rate. Differences in digestion rate have been found (at least in collagen type I) using substrate from individuals of various age. Collagen derived from diabetic patients was determined to behave like that from elderly persons. Like mammilian collagenase the clostridial collagenase is a metalloenzyme containing one zinc atom; it demands calcium for stability and is inactivated by EDTA, cysteine, or 1,10-phenylanthroline. The molecule possesses functional groups, such as carboxyl-, tyrosine-, or lysine-; blocking them inactivates the enzyme at once.

Collagenase as a Therapeutic Tool

Advancements in the understanding of the biology of healing wounds have permitted the development of surgical techniques and pharmacological agents to support and expedite the repair process. Skin wounds may be partial-thickness or full-thickness, depending upon the depth of the wound. The former will heal by reepithelization, initiated from surviving skin. The full-thickness wound involves the subcutaneous tissue and will heal either by primary or secondary intention. Healing by primary intention is simply achieved by suturing the two edges of the wound together. Healing by secondary intention is a step-by-step process involving the formation of granulation tissue, collagen formation, wound contraction, and reepithelialization.

Inhibition of the repair process may result in chronic nonhealing wounds and, as a consequence, abnormal scar formation.

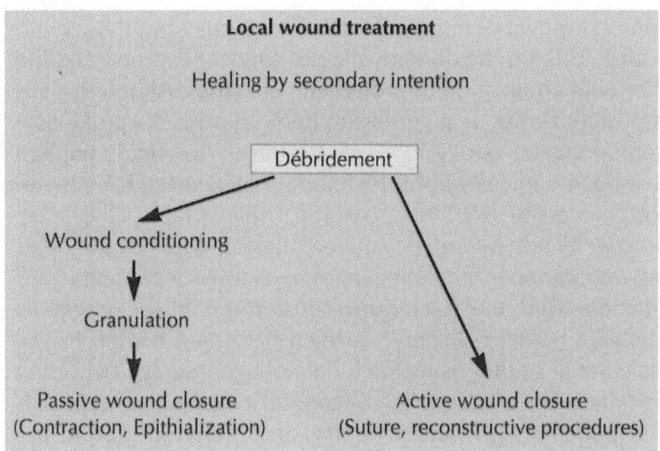

Fig. 2. Treatment design in nonhealing wounds.

Local wound treatment

Healing by secondary intention

Débridement

Wound conditioning

Granulation

Passive wound closure
(Contraction, Epithialization)

Active wound closure
(Suture, reconstructive procedures)

Retardation of tissue repair may be a result of systemic factors such as diabetes, circulatory impairment, generalized immunosuppressed states (transplant recipients, AIDS, tumor patients), or local factors such as bacterial infection and surface débris. The primary goal in the treatment of problem wounds healing by secondary intention should be rapid wound closure with good functional and cosmetic results. In order to achieve this, thorough wound débridement is the mandatory first step within a cascade of treatment modalities (Fig. 2). If wound infection is present this may be done in combination with the application of topical antimicrobials. However, such agents should not be used chronically since most of them (e.g., PVP-iodine) demonstrate cytotoxic activity, inhibiting the fibroblast proliferation necessary for ultimate wound closure and mature scar formation. Wound débridement means

Table 4. Effect of degradation of human collagens by bacterial collagenase on fibroblast chemotaxis.

Substance tested	Chemotactic activity, fibroblasts/20 OIF (mean ± SEM)
Type I	51 ± 6
Type I + collagenase	46 ± 5
Type II	57 ± 6
Type II + collagenase	45 ± 3
Type III	49 ± 4
Type III + collagenase	58 ± 5
Buffer	9 ± 1
Buffer + collagenase	7 ± 1

prompt removal of nonviable débris and pus from the wound surface. This can be done by careful surgical excision and the additional application of proteolytic enzymes. Although a variety of enzymes (e.g., trypsin-chymotrypsin, streptokinase-streptodornase, deoxyribonuclease-fibrolysin, ficin, papain) have been clinically tested, bacterial collagenase has proven most successful [19]. The reason for this is that collagenase can specifically hydrolyse native collagen, whereas the other enzymes cannot. The collagenase available for clinical use is obtained from the bacterium *Clostridium histolyticum*. Its action on native collagen has been discussed earlier. Extensive clinical studies using bacterial collagenase as a débriding agent have been undertaken by several investigators, especially in patients with burn wounds, decubitus ulcers, and peripheral vascular and diabetic ulcers [20–23]. All have shown a significant acceleration of wound healing on the basis of enhanced granulation tissue formation and epithelization. Interestingly, especially in third-degree burn wounds, the event of hypertrophic scarring and scar contracture was markedly reduced in collagenase-treated wounds [24]. Although at the moment no conclusive experimental data exist collagenase may not only expedite débridement by attacking native collagen of all types, it may also enhance macrophage chemotaxis and activation within the wound itself, thus acting to some extent as an immunmodulating agent and wound conditioner. Postlethwaite and Kang [2] have reported that macrophages and precursor monocytes, which are key promoters in the repair process, demonstrate enhanced chemotaxis upon contact with collagen-derived peptides generated by bacterial collagenase (Table 4). This same effect was shown on fibroblasts but not on neutrophils [25]. Collagen-derived peptides seem to promote granulation tissue formation by the above mechanism. Furthermore, an increase in macrophage numbers and their activation will lead to enhanced cytokine secretion in these wounds. This represents a cascade of events potentiating the immuno stimulatory effect with substantial influence on collagen formation, thus conditioning the wound for further procedures such as skin grafting.

The reason why a remarkable reduction in hypertrophic scarring is encountered in collagenase-treated wounds is not known [26, 27]. Hypertrophic scars show an increase in collagen deposition with an increase in the ratio of type-III to type-I collagen. This may be due to excessive production by activated fibroblasts or to decreased degradation by tissue collagenase. Although collagenase activity in hypertrophic scars is increased, there is evidence that the level of collagenase in-

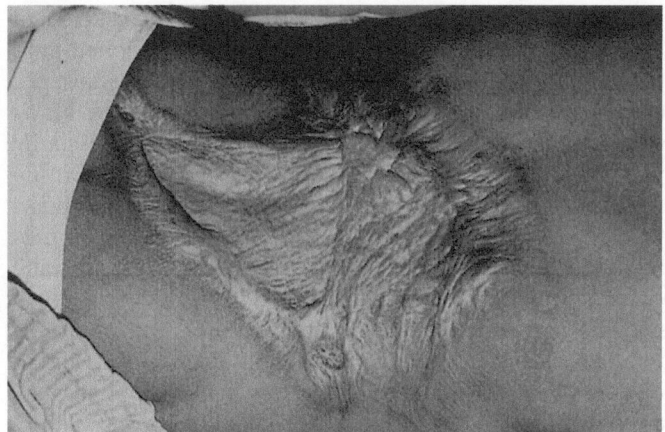

Fig. 3. Hypertrophic scar.

hibitors such as alpha-2-macroglobulin and tissue inhibitor of metalloproteinases (TIMP) is also elevated [28]. This may lead to an overall net decrease in collagen degradation with preference for certain collagen types, as has been shown in postburn wound tissues where increased collagenase activity leads to enhanced type-I collagen breakdown [9]. Bacterial collagenase degrades all types of collagen with almost the same affinity and may therefore prevent certain pathologic collagen ratios to become established, although at the moment there are no reports to support this hypothesis. Direct intradermal injection of clostridial collagenase could be promising in the treatment of hypertrophic scars and keloids. Friedman et al. [29] have shown in an experimental pig model that intradermal injection of collagenase in combination with hyaluronidase may cause dramatic degradation of dermal collagen in a dose-dependent manner, although no clinical trials have been reported to date. Further studies are needed to clarify the effect collagenase treatment of wounds has on remodeling and scar formation. However, it is an intriguing thought that selective degradation of native collagen may be a useful therapeutic tool in conditions associated with abnormal scar formation.

Conclusions

Recent advances in our understanding of basic mechanisms of wound repair have shed new light on clinical wound healing agents such as collagenase, raising new questions concerning their mode of action and possible therapeutic application. A new concept is that cells of the immune system play a dominant role in the repair process by releasing potent mediators such as cytokines and growth factors, which influence fibroblast function and angiogenesis dramatically. The first clinical trials concerning the direct application of such cloned pure growth factors have been disappointing, in that they have not yet proven superior to established treatment regimens. However, presently many studies are being undertaken to clarify their possible role as clinical woundhealing agents. On the other hand, it might be worthwhile to study old and new pharmacological substances with respect to their actions on promoter cells such as wound macrophages, which are naturally occurring production sites of those growth factors now being tested as pure preparations. It could prove more useful to modulate macrophage function, since it stands at the starting point of a whole cascade of mediators representing an intricate network of control mechanisms which are only poorly understood.

References

1. Harris ED Jr, Krane SM (1974) Collagenases (first of three parts) N Engl J Med 291:557–563
2. Postlethwaite AE, Kang AH (1976) Collagen- and collagen peptide-induced chemotaxis of human blood monocytes. J Exp Med 143:1299–1307
3. Wize J, Woitecka-Lukasik E, Maslinski S (1986) Collagen-derived peptides release mast cell histamine. Agents Actions 18:262–265
4. Postlethwaite AE, Seyer JM, Kang AH (1978) Chemotactic attraction of human fibroblasts to type I, II and III collagens and collagen-derived peptides. Proc Natl Acad Sci USA 75:871–875
5. Craig P (1973) Collagenase activity in cutaneous scars. Hand 5:239–246
6. Dresden MH, Heilmann SA, Schmidt JD (1972) Collagenolytic enzymes in human neoplasms. Cancer Res 32:993–996
7. Liotta LA, Tyggvason K, Gorbisa S, Hart J, Foltz CM, Shafie S (1980) Metastatic potential correlates with enzymatic degradation of basement membrane collagen. Nature 284:67–68
8. Young HC, Wheeler MH (1983) Collagenase inhibition in the healing colon, J R Soc Med 76:32–36
9. Kishi K, Hashimoto Y, Aoyama H, Izawa Y, Hayakawa T (1984) Direct extraction of collagenase from human post-burn wound tissues. Biomed Res 5:149–156
10. Grillo HC, Gross J (1967) Collagenolytic activity during mammalian wound repair. Dev Biol 15:300–317
11. Black CT, Hennessey PJ, Ford EG, Andrassy RJ (1989) Protein glycosylation and collagen metabolism in normal and diabetic rats. J Surg Res 47:200–202
12. Mallya SK, Mookhtiar KA, Gao Y, Brew K, Dioszegi M, Birkedal-Hansen H, van Wart HE (1990) Characterization of 58-kilodalton human neutrophil collagenase: comparison with human fibroblast collagenase. Biochemistry 29:10628–10634
13. Birkedal-Hansen B, Moore WGI, Taylor RE, Bhown AS, Birkedal-Hansen H (1988) Monoclonal antibodies to human fibroblast collagenase. Inhibition of enzymatic activity, affinity purification of the enzyme and

evidence for clustering of epitopes in the NH_2-terminal end of the activated enzyme. Biochemistry 27:6751–6758

14. Dayer J-M, Stephenson ML, Schmidt E, Karge W, Krane SM (1981) Purification of a factor from human blood monocyte-macrophages, which stimulates the production of collagenase and PGE_2 by cells cultured from rheumathoid synovial tissues. FEBS Lett 124:253

15. Postlethwaite AE, Lachman LB, Mainardi CL, Kang AH (1983) Interleukin 1 stimulation of collagenase production by cultured fibroblasts. J Exp Med 157:801–806

16. Bauer EA, Cooper TW, Huang JS, Altman J, Deuel TF (1985) Stimulation in vitro of human skin collagenase expression by platelet-derived growth fractor. Proc Natl Acad Sci USA 82:4132–4136

17. Macartney HW, Tschesche H (1981) A metal ion requirement for activation of latent collagenase from human PMNLs. Hoppe-Seylers Z Physiol Chem 362:1523–1531

18. Keil B (1988) Recent development in the research of structure-function relationships in collagenases. Pathol Biol 36: 1112–1118

19. Boxer AM, Gottesman N, Bernstein H, Mandl I (1969) Débridement of dermal ulcers and decubitus with collagenase. Geriatrics 24:75–86

20. Lee LK, Ambrus JL (1975) Collagenase therapy for decubitus ulcers. Geriatrics 30:91–98

21. Varma AO, Bugatch E, Gemram FM (1973) Débridement of dermal ulcers with collagenase. Surg Gynecol Obstet 136:281–282

22. Paul E (1990) Wundheilung unter Iruxol. Fortschr Med 35: 679–681

23. Blum G (1973) Therapeutische Erfahrungen mit Iruxol bei Ulcera cruris, Dekubitus und Verbrennungen. Schweiz Rundsch Med Prax 62:820–826

24. Purder K (1973) Erfahrungsbericht über die Anwendung von Iruxol Salbe bei Verbrennungen. Z Allgemeinmed 49: 856–858

25. Albini A, Adelmann-Grill BC (1985) Collagenolytic cleavage products of collagen type I as chemoattractants for human dermal fibroblasts. Eur J Cell Biol 36:104–107

26. Diegelmann RF, Bryant CP, Cohen IK (1977) Tissue alpha-globulins in keloid formation. Plast Reconstr Surg 59:418–423

27. Cohen IK, Diegelmann PF, Keiser HR (1973) Collagen metabolism in keloid and hypertrophic scar. In: Longacre JJ (ed) The ultrastructure of collagen. Thomas, Springfield, pp 199–212

28. Hembry RM, Ehrlich HP (1986) Immunolocalization of collagenase and tissue inhibitor of metalloproteinases (TIMP) in hypertrophic scar tissue. Br J Dermatol 115:409–420

29. Friedman K, Pollack SV, Manning T, Pinell SR (1986) Degradation of porcine dermal connective tissue by collagenase and hyaluronidase. Br J Dermatol 115:403–408

Interview

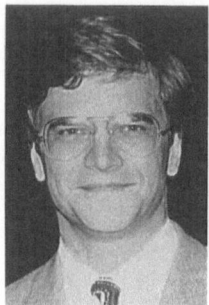

Can you tell us something about your scientific work with collagenases?
Hatz: In our laboratory at the University of Munich we have been working with collagenase for the past two years. We have been particularly interested in the immune mechanisms that collagenase might affect following application of the enzyme on healing wounds.

How can collagenase influence scarring?
Hatz: Interestingly, the scar tissue which forms following collagenase treatement is quite different from that which results from normal wound healing. In a hypertrophic scar collagen III dominates over collagen I. The normal scar has more collagen I than collagen III. Actually we are very interested in finding out why collagenase treatment prevents hypertrophic scarring. We would like to show that the ratio of collagen can be changed by applying collagenase in the direction of more type I collagen.

What is the effect of topical collagenase on a wound?
Hatz: In chronic wounds like decubitus and leg ulcers, the level of collagenase is low. Applying collagenase here helps the natural process. Collagenase digests collagen into small fragments, which can attract macrophages and neutrophils. This is how collagenase might influence repair mechanisms in the early phase of wound healing. The other aspect is a change in the ratio of type III to type I collagen.

Collagenase, Aid for Treatment of Decubitus Ulcers

M. W. F. van Leen

Summary

Despite optimal preventive measures it is impossible to fully eliminate factors that could lead to a decubitus ulcer. In these wounds it is often not possible to surgically remove the necrosis without damaging healthy tissue. In a multicenter study, 63 inpatients with decubitus ulcers grade III or IV were treated with collagenases once daily for 8 weeks; 60% of the patients had a clean wound after 2–4 weeks. The decrease of inflammatory symptoms was significant and alleviated the discomfort of the patients. This acceleration of the wound healing results in a quicker recovery of the patients and is therefore cost saving.

Introduction

The best way to treat decubitus ulcers is to prevent them from forming. Despite optimum preventive actions, however, it is impossible to fully eliminate factors that can lead to decubitus. In recent years attention has been drawn to prevention, especially in hospitals, during operations or long-term immobilization.

With every decubitus ulcer, necrotic tissue forms which adheres to the healthy tissue via collagen fibrils. Wound cure can be achieved only if necrotic tissue is fully rejected. A swift and most effective method for removing necrosis is surgical necrotomy. Unfortunately, in the case of decubitus ulcers it is often impossible to treat the necrosis in such a manner without damaging healthy tissue. The treatment of the remnants is generally performed with the aid of proteolytic enzymes.

A well-known enzyme, capable of removing unchanged collagen tissue, is collagenase [2, 3, 6, 7, 9, 12–14]. The body's own collagenases are secreted by fibroblasts, keratinocytes, macrophages, and granulocytes. Certain body substances

Verpleeghuis de Naaldhorst, Middelbroekweg, 2671 ME Naaldwijk, NL such as interleukin 1, prostaglandin E_2 and some immuno-globulins are responsible for the increase of the synthesis of collagenases.

From studies performed in the United States [1], Switzerland [8], Germany [10, 11] and Italy [4], it appears that addition of the collagenases obtained from the culture of the bacterium *Clostridium histolyticum* leads to speedy wound recovery. The basic enzyme, clostridiopeptidase A, splits only the native collagen, by means of which necrotic material is broken down and removed. Accompanying proteases which arise during the production of clostridiopeptidase A are responsible for the nonspecific breakdown of protein and therefore take care of the removal of other albuminous material.

Materials and Study Plan

A multicenter trial in nine nursing homes throughout the Netherlands included a total of 63 inpatients (45 women and 18 men). The average age was 76.3 years (range, 45–93). The inclusion criteria were decubitus grade III or IV with necrosis, age more than 18 years, and signing of informed consent. The exclusion criteria were serious wound infections, combination with other proteolytic enzymes, ointment with heavy metals, and/or allergy for collagenases.

At the start and end of the study a medical examination was conducted to evaluate the general state of health, mental state, mobility, incontinence, intake of fluid and nutrition, and predisposing diseases (Knoll scale, see Table 1). The decubitus ulcer was judged at the start and thereafter once a week for a maximum of 8 weeks (minimum 4 weeks) with regard to size, depth, signs of inflammation (redness, exudate, and pain), area of necrosis, presence of granulation, epithelialization, and yellow slough. The wound borders were checked for maceration, eczema, and itching. Also once a week a color picture of the wound was taken. At the start and end of the study a basic laboratory workup was also conducted.

The wound treatment consisted of cleaning and/or moistening the bed of the wound with NaCl 0.9%. Collagenase[1] was applied in a 1- to 2-mm layer and covered with paraffin gauze and an absorbent bandage. The paraffin gauze fully covered the wound borders. Wounds were treated once a day. If possible a surgical necrotomy was conducted prior to the study; this was not allowed during the study.

---

[1] Collagenase 1.2 units/g in lipophilic anhydrous ointment base.

Table 1. Knoll Scale.

I	General state of health		
		good	0
		fair	1
		poor	2
		moribund	3
II	Mental status		
		alert	0
		lethargic	1
		semicomatose	2
		comatose	3
III	Activity		
		ambulatory	0
		needs help	1
		in wheelchair	4
		bedridden	6
IV	Mobility		
		full	0
		limited	1
		very limited	4
		immobile	6
V	Incontinence (urinary)		
		absent	0
		occasional	1
		frequent	4
		total	6
VI	Nutritional status		
	Oral nutrition intake		
		good (> 1500 kcal)	0
		fair (1000–1500 kcal)	1
		poor (500–1000 kcal)	2
		none (< 500 kcal)	3
	Oral fluid intake		
		good (> 1500 ml)	0
		fair (1000–1500 ml)	1
		poor (500–1000 ml)	2
		none (< 500 cc)	3
VII	Predisposing diseases		
		absent	0
		slight	1
		moderate	2
		severe	3

Results

Of the 63 patients 43 were evaluable. Twenty did not comply with the demands of the protocol. Within 4 weeks after the start, 13 patients died of causes unrelated to the use of collagenase. Two patients had to be admitted and with five the attending physician found it necessary to adjust the treatment, which was not allowed by the protocol.

For this group the score according to the Knoll scale was higher and increased until the time of death or termination of the study. For patients who terminated the study the Knoll scale did not change and averaged 9.8 on a scale of maximally 33 points (Table 1).

At the start of the treatment there were 47 patients with more than 50% and 16 with less than 50% of the wound surface

Table 2. Wound cleaning.

	Percent	Cumulative percent
After 1–2 weeks	9.8	9.8
After 2–4 weeks	51.2	61.0
After 4–6 weeks	12.2	73.2
After 6–8 weeks	17.1	90.2
Nonresponders	9.8	100.0

Table 3. Difference after treatment in wound size, wound depth, area of necrosis, granulation, yellow slough, signs of inflammation, and wound borders for all patients who completed the study.

		Female	Male	All
Size of ulcer	Mean	0.48	0.20	0.33
	P-value	0.0	0.44	0.01
Wound depth	Mean	0.39	0.30	0.37
	P-value	0.03	0.19	0.01
Area of necrosis	Mean	0.52	0.30	0.47
	P-value	0.00	0.08	0.00
Granulation	Mean	0.70	0.40	0.63
	P-value	0.00	0.17	0.00
Epithelialization	Mean	0.76	0.60	0.72
	P-value	0.00	0.01	0.01
Yellow slough	Mean	0.30	0.00	0.23
	P-value	0.01	1.00	0.02
Signs of inflammation	Mean	1.39	1.30	1.37
	P-value	0.00	0.06	0.00
Wound borders	Mean	0.06	0.30	0.02
	P-value	0.66	0.19	0.84
Duration of treatment	Mean	6.48	5.60	6.28
	S.D.	1.79	1.78	1.80

Table 4. Start of granulation.		
	Percent	Cumulative percent
After 1–2 weeks	13.9	13.9
After 2–4 weeks	69.4	83.3
After 4–8 weeks	5.6	88.9
Nonresponders	11.1	100.0

covered with necrosis. The average treatment period was 6 weeks. With 61% of the patients the necrosis was removed after 4 weeks, with 73.2% after 6 weeks. With 10% there were no positive results after 8 weeks (Table 2).

Table 3 details differences in wound characteristics. Wound size, wound depth surface of necrosis, and yellow slough decreased significantly ($P = 0.01$). One of the most important experiences was that all inflammation symptoms (redness, exudate, and pain) diminished. The signs of inflammation individually and statistically improved significantly ($P = 0.01$). Increase of granulation and epithelialization were statistically significant ($P = 0.01$). The changes in the wound borders were not statistically significant. The wound size of patients who reacted to the treatment diminished. Wound size was exclusively observed as surface. Unfortunately, an accurate three-dimensional determination was lacking in all institutions.

At the start of the study the subject of granulation tissue had not yet been broached. The development of granulation tissue appeared after 2 weeks in 80% of the patients (see Table 4). As far as can be judged, there was no reason for a delayed development of granulation tissue. Studies performed in Munich have confirmed this phenomenon [5]. No allergic or toxic reactions appeared. Worsening of pain was not indicated by the patients. The combination of collagenases with paraffin did not cause maceration of the wound borders.

Discussion and Conclusion

Decubitus ulcers are a serious and frequent complication after long-term low pressure or brief high pressure and/or shearing forces, especially among elderly people. They cause much pain and many hygienic problems for the patient. Therefore, wound treatment serves as aim to shorten the duration and to ease the pain. A side from treatment products and preventive

Fig. 1a–c
Decubitus ulcer
a before,
b 7 days after and
c 21 days after treatment with collagenase 1,2

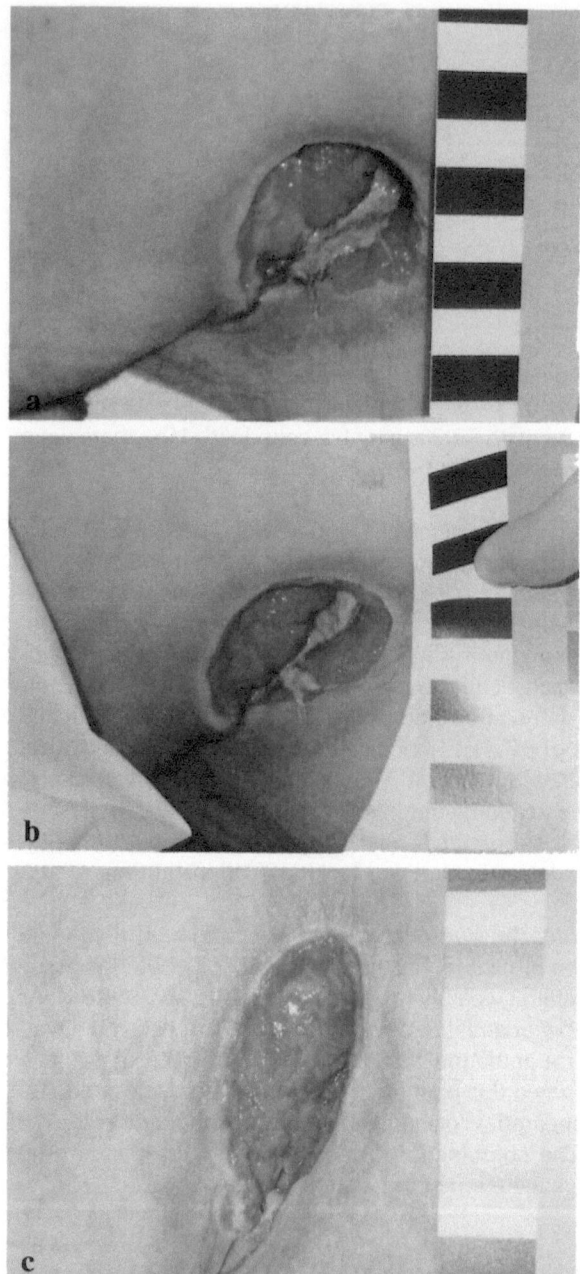

materials, wound treatment is also labor intensive. Speeding up the wound cleaning will result in a quicker recovery and is therefore cost saving. Previous studies have indicated that addition of collagenases will bring about faster wound cleaning.

Table 5. Evaluation of treatment.

	Percent	Cumulative percent
Very good	7.3	7.3
Good	68.3	75.6
Moderate	14.6	90.2
Nonresponders	9.8	100.0

This study has shown that 60% of the patients had a clean wound after 2–4 weeks. A once-a-day application of Collagenase, without protection of the wound borders and covering with paraffin gauze, seems a huge gain for the present wound cleaning of necrosis. Protective ointment on the wound borders was not necessary. Through decrease of inflammation symptoms the comfort of the patients improved. Seventy-five percent of the researchers were satisfied with the results of the trial (Table 5).

Interesting is the phenomenon that with the use of collagenases granulation tissue formation and epithelialization remain a possibility.

Since special types of collagenases could accelerate epithelialization [5] I questioned at what stage of the wound healing the use of *Collagenase ointment* should be stopped. A pilot study including five patients with whom *Collagenase ointment* had been continued revealed complete healing of the wound. Therefore, I am of the opinion that this is reason for a further study.

Acknowledgements. I wish to express my appreciation to the doctors and nurses in the nursing homes included: *St. Jozefzorg*-Tilburg, *Huize Westhoff*-Rijswijk, *De Blinkert*-Baarn, *Coendershof*-Groningen, *Solwerd*-Appingedam, *Clara Feyoena Heem*-Hardenberg, *Stichting Verzorging Verpleging Revalidatie*-Zoetermeer, Nicolaas Nursing Home-Lutjebroek and Nursing Home De Naaldhorst-Naaldwijk.

I also thank Leo Sahelijo, Edgar Geervliet, and Jim Tolsma of Knoll for providing the materials, as well as for their support, and my secretary, Marian Flaton, for her cooperation and her patience.

References

1. Rao DB et al. (1975) Collagenase in the treatment of dermal and decubitus ulcers. J Am Geriatr Soc 22–30
2. Margulis RR et al (1961) Use of proteolytic enzymes in surgical complications. A J Obstet Gynecol 81:840–847
3. Stüwe U (1983) Enzymatische Wundreinigung. Fortschr Med 101: 1883–1888
4. Palmieri B et al (1992) Collagenase mono ointment vs. placebo in the treatment of ulcers of the lower extremities, a double-blind study. European Congress on Wound Healing and Skin Physiology, Bochum
5. Hatz RA et al (1992) Mechanisms of action of collagenase in wound repair. European Congress on Wound Healing and Skin Physiology, Bochum
6. Beatriz H et al (1991) Collagenase production at the border of granulation tissue in a healing wound: macrophage and mesenchynal collagenase production in vivo. Connective Tissue Res 27:63–71
7. Boxer AM et al (1967) Débridement of dermal ulcers and decubiti with collagenase. Geriatrics 24–27, 75–86
8. Helali P et al (1980) Chirurgische Wundheilungsstörungen und enzymatische Therapie mit einer Kollagenase-Präparation. Schweiz Rundsch Med Prax 69:703–711
9. Lee LK et al (1975) Collagenase therapy for decubitus ulcers. Geriatrics 30:91–98
10. Anonymous (1989) Doppelblindstudie zur Prüfung der wundreinigenden Wirkung von Novuxol vs. Salbengrundlage. Knoll AG, Ludwigshafen
11. Paul E (1990) Wundheilung unter Iruxol. Fortschr Med 109:NR 35–1990
12. Vanscheidt W (1992) Wundheilungsstörungen: Beilage für Hautärzte. Springer, Berlin Heidelberg New York
13. Zucearelli GC et al (1990) Collagenase in the treatment of decubitus ulcers in elderly high-risk patients. Giron Gerontol 38:237–241
14. Varma AO et al (1973) Débridement of dermal ulcers with collagenase. Surg Gynaecol Obstet 136:281

Interview

What is best therapeutic approach to decubitus?
van Leen: The best way to treat pressure sores is, of course, to prevent them. If a pressure sore has developed, wound cure can be achieved if necrotic tissue is fully rejected. Surgical necrotomy is unfortunately often not able to treat necrosis in such a manner without damaging healthy tissue. Most of the wounds will retain some necrotic tissue which adheres to the healthy tissue by collagen fibrils. The addition of collagenases will effect a more rapid wound cleaning.

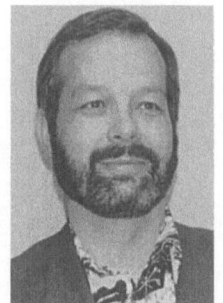

What kind of clinical research on pressure sores did you perform?
van Leen: Based on a study with collagenase by Palmieri in Italy, we conducted a multicenter study in nine nursing homes throughout the Netherlands. The inclusion criteria were decubitus grade III or IV with necrosis.

Can you give some more details about the study performance?
van Leen: The patients were observed for at least 4 weeks. Wound treatment took place once a day. We cleaned the wound with NaCl 0.9%. Collagenase was applied in a 1- to 2-mm layer and covered with paraffin gauze and an absorbent bandage. During the study necrotomy was not allowed.

What are the main results of your study?
van Leen: A total of 43 patients with pressure sores were evaluated. No allergic or toxic reactions were observed. Worsening of pain was not indicated by the patients either. Sixty percent of the patients had a clean wound after 2–4 weeks. Remarkable were a decrease of inflammatory signs like redness, exudate, and pain and a continuation of granulation and epithelialization in the decubitus wounds.

Future Prospects of Proteolytic Enzymes and Wound Healing

W. Westerhof

A review of the literature makes it clear that the effects of the various proteolytic enzymes presently on the market have not been sufficiently investigated in double-blind placebo-controlled clinical trials. This is primarily because most of these enzyme preparations were introduced a long time ago, when the regulations of the health authorities were not very strict. Furthermore, the evaluation methods and end-point criteria for a clinical study were not very accurate. Finally, most of the studies suffered a lack of stratification, involving huge numbers of patients, mostly in poorly organized multi center trials. This is now going to change. The Food and Drug Administration of the USA and the Committee for Proprietary Medicinal Products of the FC have set very strict guidelines on the quality, safety, and efficacy of medicinal products for human use. This means that many existing products have to be filed again for registration according to the new guidelines of good clinical, laboratory, and manufacturing practice.

With the advent of computer image analysis techniques, it is now possible to evaluate processes of wound healing and necrotic tissue débridement very accurately [1, 2]. This also automatically results in smaller numbers of patients to be investigated which can be performed in one center, involving one trial doctor. This all means fewer variables and greater reliability [3]. In vitro models and animal models can, of course, in the preclinical phase elucidate the efficacy and safety of an enzyme preparation [4, 5]. The choice of the animal model is thereby of eminent importance. We think that the necrotic wound model in the pig comes closest to the human situation [6]. This model can also be used for dose-finding studies.

Apart from testing the efficacy of the existing products, it would also be attractive to study new enzyme preparations [7]. The list of enzymes recovered from plants and animals is

Department of Dermatology, Academic Medical Center, University of Amsterdam, The Netherlands still growing [8]. Knowing their substrate specificity it is possible to develop preparations which might be more selective and more efficient in breaking down necrotic tissue. In this respect it is necessary to know exactly the molecular composition of the extracellular matrix (ECM) and the cell membranes of cells in various tissues such as skin, bones, and internal organs.

Some enzymes can act only when they are not in solution, but rather immobilized on a membrane [9]. This offers possibilities of combining enzyme preparations with other solid wound products to create a combination product. Granulate materials or gels are most suitable, as these application forms guarantee optimal contact with the surface of the necrotic wound. The advantage of using immobilized enzymes is that autodigestion does not take place at the same speed as when they are present in solution, so that enzymes of different backgrounds can be used in combination.

Apart from the strictly proteolytic effect, it is also necessary to investigate the effect of proteolytic enzymes in other biological aspects of wound healing [10]. One group of proteolytic enzymes are the proteases, which are capable of splitting proteins but are also able to bind to cell receptors, e.g., fibroblasts, resulting in cell proliferation [11].

In 1970 the growth-stimulating property was described for pronase, ficin, and trypsin [12]. In the wound itself metalloproteinases are synthesized e.g., collagenase, which breaks down collagen, thus making the migration of fibroblasts possible [13]. It is not clear whether collagenase can also induce cell proliferation; however, this has been shown for thrombin.

Sometimes, through the action of enzyme breakdown products of the ECM, components fulfill some of the criteria described for wound angiogenic factors e.g. degradation of macromolecular hyaluronan by enzymes [14].

It is also possible that the cleansing effect of krill enzymes may lead to the generation of in situ growth factors by alarmed neighboring cells, or to molecular remnants produced by the proteolytic cleavage of tissue matrix into fragments. These, in turn, can act either as chemotactic factors for immunocompetent cells or directly, as the stimulating agents on keratinocytes, endothelial cells, and fibroblasts. In other words, the generation of granulation tissue by enzymes may be an indirect consequence of their cleansing effect on the skin as a whole organ. Therefore, it remains possible that certain enzymes constitutively exert a mitogenic effect in skin as a whole tissue, rather than on separate cell monocultures. However, the overall pathophysiological steps involved in wound healing cannot be studied collectively using the histiotypic culture of individual cells [4]. The organotypic culture model offers an attractive alternative system, which can mimic living skin [5]. The use of this model to investigate the conditions affecting epidermal growth and differentiation is well documented.

Through the better understanding of the (inter)action of proteolytic enzymes in wound healing and wound débridement it is envisaged that more efficient, selective, and safe products will be developed. With the close interaction of industrial laboratories, academic research groups, and clinicians these developments can be tested and put into practice.

References

1. Hellgren L, Vincent J (1993) Evaluation techniques for the assessment of wound healing. In: Westerhof W (ed) Leg ulcers: diagnosis and treatment, Elsevier Science Publishers Amsterdam, pp 381–384
2. Mekkes JR, Westerhof W, van Rietpaap E, Estevez O (1993) A new computer image analysis system designed for evaluating wound débriding products. In: Proc. of meeting on advances in wound management (Oktober 20–23 1992, Harrogate, Harding KG et al. (eds). MacMillan Magazines, London, pp 4–7
3. Westerhof W, Mekkes JR, Le Poole IC, Das PK (1993) Research on leg ulcers. In: Westerhof W (ed) Leg ulcers: diagnosis and treatment. Elsevier Science Publishers, Amsterdam, pp 385–399
4. Le Poole IC, Das PK, Krieg SR, Mekkes JR, Westerhof W (1991) Organotypic culture of human skin for studying wound healing. Wounds 3:102–110
5. Le Poole IC, Das PK, Dingemans KP, de Boer OJ, Boschman GA, Mekkes JR, Westerhof W (1990) In vitro effect of "krill enzymes" on skin cell types related to wound healing. Wounds 2:163–169
6. Mekkes JR, Westerhof W, Le Poole IC, Das PK (1990) Proteolytic débridement of necrotic wounds using krill enzymes in a pig model. J Invest Dermatol 95:480
7. Westerhof W, Mekkes JR (1990) Krill and other enzymes in enzymatic wound débridement. In: Wadström T et al. (eds) Pathogenesis of wound and biomaterial-associated infections. Springer, Berlin Heidelberg New York, pp 179–188
8. Dixon M et al (1984) International Union of Biochemistry (Nomenclature Committee). Enzyme Nomenclature 1984. Academic, London
9. Mosback K (1976) *Immobilized enzymes* appeared in *Methods in enzymology*. vol XLIV. Academic, New York
10. Dutrieux RP, Van Ginkel CJW, Westerhof W (1989) Toepassing van groeifactoren bij wondgenezing: fictie of realiteit? Ned Tijdschr Geneesk 133:1870–1872
11. Sher W (1987) The role of extracellular proteases in cell proliferation and differentiation. Lab Invest 57:607–633

12. Burger M (1970) Proteolytic enzymes initiating cell division and escape from contact inhibition of growth. Nature 227:170–171
13. Kodama S, Kishi J, Obata K, Iwata K, Hayakawa T (1987) Monoclonal antibodies to bovine inhibitor. Coll Relat Res 7:341–350
14. Nakamura T, Takagaki K, Kubo K, Morikawa A, Tamura S, Endo M (1990) Extracellular depolymerisation of hyaluronic acid in cultured human skin fibroblasts. Biochem Biophys Res Commun 172:70–76

Subject Index

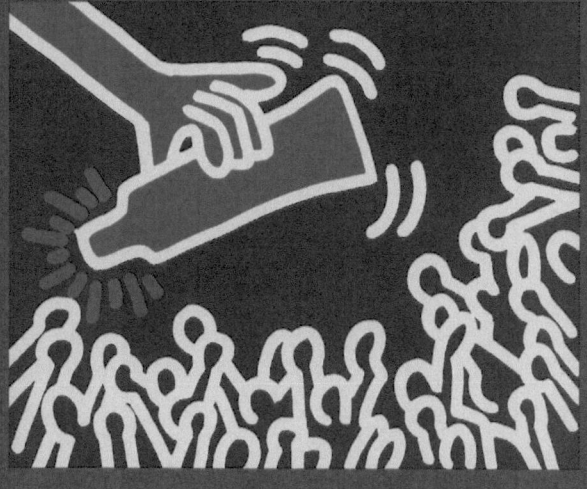